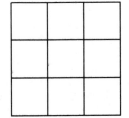

Successful STYLE

**A MAN'S GUIDE TO
A COMPLETE PROFESSIONAL IMAGE**

Successful
STYLE

DORIS POOSER

CRISP PUBLICATIONS, INC.

To The Memory Of
James Elliott Pooser.

Successful Style:
A Man's Guide to a Complete Professional Image
by Doris Pooser

Published by
Crisp Publications, Inc.
95 First Street
Los Altos, CA 94022
(415) 949-4888

Art Direction & Design by Robert Hickey,
  Aubergine Communications
Illustration by April Reinking
Author Photo by Lisa Mason

ACKNOWLEDGMENTS

●●

I am often asked how long it takes to write a book like Successful Style. Any project of this size is the result of a lifetime of experiences. These experiences, good and bad, provide the opportunity to develop, create and test concepts that can eventually be put into words. From the first drop of ink on the paper until the final book rolls off the press, the project becomes a team effort. Each player on the team is important and deserves special thanks.

I want to thank the Always In Style consultants, staff and friends who enthusiastically supported the project.

Special thanks are in order for many:

Angie Michael, Director of Training for Always In Style, and as a contributing editor working with me to expand and develop content material.

Phil Trupp for his major contribution in writing, and editing.

Mary Zimmerman, Kathy Kienke, Joy Mahovich, Bonny Barshay, Bonnie Miller, Mary Jane Barnes, Louise Wiltshire, Rebecca Giles-Wiltshire, and Jean Gaffney who worked with Angie Michael to test the material and offer recommendations based on their experiences as the top image consultants in the nation.

Val Gardner for line editing of the manuscript.

Robert Hickey, Art Director, for his organizational skills, ideas and ongoing support.

Wanda Little Fenimore, Beth Baldwin, Cindy Cooper, Gus Costas, Don Watts and Gentry Ferrell for their coordination and hard work behind the scenes.

HDL publishers, especially Chuck Durang and Richard Re, for the opportunity to work with such professional entrepreneurs who are positive, supportive and enthusiastic.

Lastly to Todd and Jeoffrey Pooser, my two sons, for their love, support, and dedication that enabled me to complete this project and to begin once again and to look ahead.

DORIS POOSER
ACCOLADE, INC.

CONTENTS

●●

Basic corporate, off-hour and casual wardrobes.
Formal wear. Putting a basic wardrobe plan in action.

Basic looks for all occasions.

The difference between fashion and styles.
Understanding your face and body shapes. How to match
clothing and body lines. Easy guidelines for selecting
suits and shirts. The best hairstyle and eyeglass frames
for your face shape.

MEMO

●●●

TO:
PROFESSIONALS ON
THE WAY TO THE TOP

Successful Style is for men who know that style counts!

Style really does. Attend a board meeting anywhere in the world. The men seated around the table may be different when it comes to ideas, ambition, drive, or their tastes. But they all share a desire to look great. Which is one of the reasons they are where they are — at the top.

As president of Accolade, Inc., I work with men from the boardroom to the mailroom. Many are at the top of their professions — and still the need to know, to fine-tune their style is a constant.

It has little, if anything, to do with vanity. Great style does more than impart a feeling of well-being. It's a vital element of self confidence and in business it pays handsome dividends.

Recently, Accolade held a series of seminars for State Farm Insurance, one of the biggest corporations in America. Our mission was to define style and relate it to the executives, individually. It produced some eye-opening results.

I asked a group of executives to come on stage to help in an experiment. Just by looking at them, I told them I could choose the most senior and successful man, "The man from whom I'd buy insurance," I told them confidently.

Six volunteered. I scanned each and picked the last gentleman in the group, the one I'd trust with my own insurance needs. He turned out to be the president.

I had no advance knowledge, yet the president looked the part. His appearance projected confidence, taste, power, ease.

One of his executives was a bit shaken and said, "What's so different about the way I look compared to him?"

He asked for it, so I pointed to his double-knit jacket which was too cozy for his body, the too-short necktie, his "high-water" trousers, the shoes that matched nothing else, and the white socks. In comparison, his boss wore a well-tailored suit; his shirt and necktie were perfectly combined, and it was clear he had a careful eye for the right colors. Everything about him said "success."

This isn't to suggest that appearance is everything. But one thing is certain: *If you look as if you belong at the top, chances are you're already there or on the way!*

Obviously, ideas about style, taste, and grooming have a way of becoming blurred by opinions. We've avoided this trap. *Successful Style* is based on solid data and what our Always In Style consultants have learned working with men all over the world. What you'll find in these pages has statistical depth. If we offer an opinion, we say so; otherwise, we draw directly from our universe of clients.

Our focus is on your "total presentation" — the mix of verbal and non-verbal signals. In the professional world it's axiomatic that people who make positive impressions non-verbally (looking great), and who follow up with a strong verbal presentation are more confident, get the best breaks, and are in a position to shift the odds of success in their favor.

Successful Style comes to you with a promise: To help you develop your style and total presentation in an easy, uncluttered, step-by-step way. If you're going to make it to the top — and stay there — this book is your passport to success.

DORIS POOSER
ACCOLADE, INC.

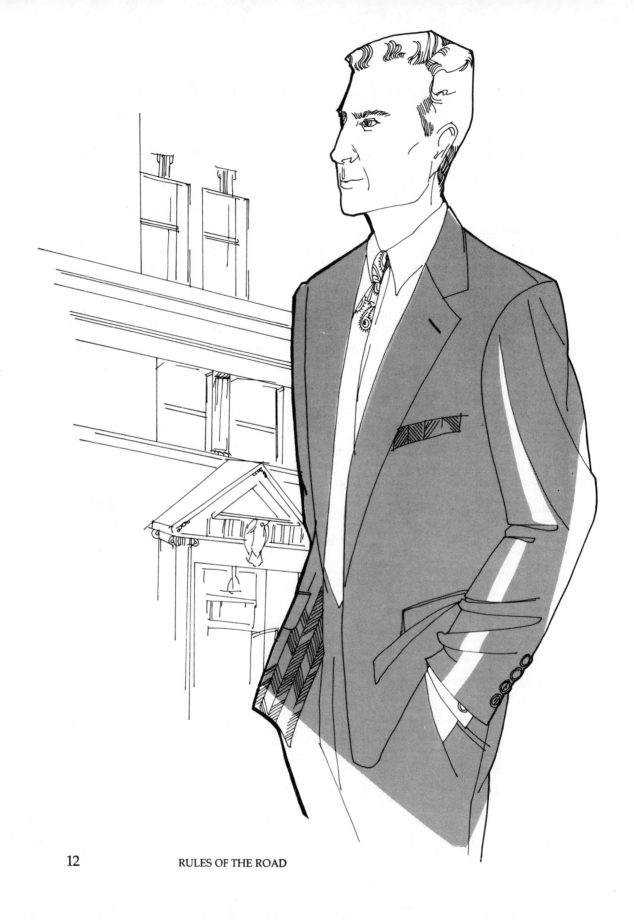

RULES OF THE ROAD

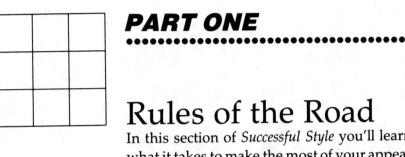

PART ONE

●●●●●●●●●●●●●●●●●●●●●●●●●●●●●●●●●●●●

Rules of the Road

In this section of *Successful Style* you'll learn the ABC's of what it takes to make the most of your appearance and how to craft your own special style.

The basics, outlined in Chapter One, will provide you with a basic wardrobe plan for business, leisure, and important formal occasions.

You'll also learn how to personalize your wardrobe so that it heightens your strong points and minimizes weaknesses.

I want to emphasize that the skills are based on solid, time-tested methods; *they are not a collection of vague opinions, fads, or fancies.* There is a definite science behind the "art" of personal appearance, and this, as much as possible, will be your guide.

At the end of each chapter you'll find a checklist to test your knowledge and affirm the rules of the road.

Keep in mind that the principles of personal style are much less subjective than you might have imagined. Those discussed here have worked for thousands of men; they are *empirical and can be tested.* After all, if your appearance is critical to success in your professional and personal life, it's far too important to be left to feelings or iffy concepts of taste. Making it to the top isn't a guessing game.

I believe you'll find these rules of the road to be exciting and rewarding. Being the best you can be is an adventure of self-discovery, and that's really the goal — to discover those personal qualities that lend to self-confidence, satisfaction, and the highest rewards.

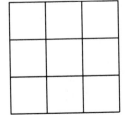

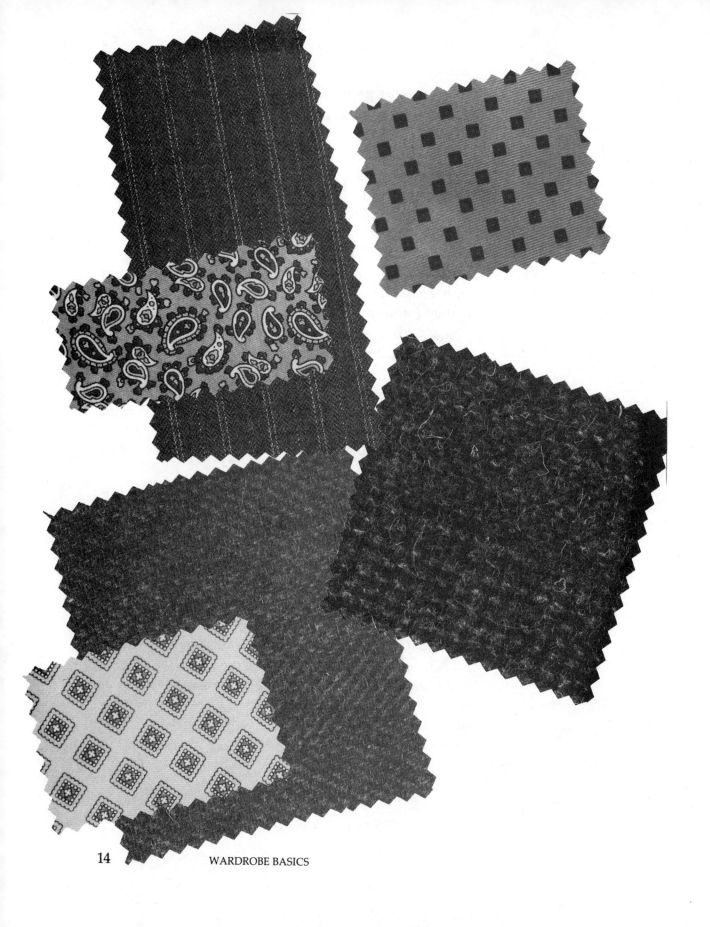

14   WARDROBE BASICS

CHAPTER ONE

WARDROBE BASICS

To succeed at anything worthwhile you need a basic plan — a plan that's right for you and is custom-made for your needs.

In this chapter we'll outline three rock-bottom wardrobe plans, essentially the minimum items you'll need for business, casual, or leisure wear, and the extras you can use to make the most of formal occasions.

The plans are based on a survey of hundreds of executives and professionals operating in a wide spectrum of business environments, from entrepreneurial start-ups to "mega-corps" such as Xerox and General Motors. The executives surveyed were asked to list their basic working wardrobes, including number of suits, shirts, neckties, shoes, and other items they deemed absolutely essential to their activities at work and during their off-hours. We averaged the numbers and came up with the following:

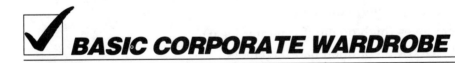 **BASIC CORPORATE WARDROBE**

☐ **Suits:**
- Gray suit (solid)
- Navy suit (solid)
- Pin stripe or chalk stripe suit

The three suits listed above are considered critical to the demands of the daily working environment. Later, most executives add two more offerings:

- A patterned suit (Glenn plaid or herringbone)
- An additional color, something other than gray or navy or a combination such as a tweed or tone-on-tone.

☐ **Dress shirts:**
- Five white shirts
- Five blue shirts
- Three striped shirts
- Five colors, usually beige, pink, yellow, or pearl gray

☐ **Neckties:**
- Two solids
- Five striped
- Three foulard
- Two dots
- Three paisley and/or club ties

☐ **Shoes:**
- One pair lace-ups or tassel loafers (dark color)
- Two pairs of plain-toed slip-ons (dark color — and *not moccasins*)

☐ **Belts:**
- Two high-quality leather belts (dark)

☐ **Socks:**
- One dozen pairs solid color (dark)

☐ **Coats:**
- One raincoat or trench coat (tan)
- One overcoat or top coat

☐ **Accessories:**
- One scarf (wool or cashmere)
- Good leather briefcase (no exaggerated combination locks)
- Umbrella (dark)
- Watch (good quality, non-digital)
- Leather gloves (high quality for winter wear)
- One dozen cotton or linen handkerchiefs

BUILDING A BASIC CORPORATE WARDROBE

Basic Business Wardrobe	My Actual Wardrobe	Items I Need in My Wardrobe
SUITS - 3 TO 5		
1 gray		
1 navy		
1 pin stripe or chalk-stripe		
2 optional patterns or colors		
SHIRTS - 15		
5 white		
5 blue		
3 striped		
4 colors: beige, pink, yellow or pearl grey		
TIES - 15 TO 20		
2 solids		
4 striped		
4 foulard		
3 dots		
2 paisley and/ or club ties		
SHOES -3		
1 pair lace-ups black		
2 pair of plain-toed slip-ons: black or dark color		
BELTS -2		
2 dark leather		

For more details, see the text in this chapter.

BUILDING A BASIC CORPORATE WARDROBE

Basic Business Wardrobe	My Actual Wardrobe	Items I Need in My Wardrobe
SOCKS - 12		
1 dozen pairs dark solid colors	_____	_____
	_____	_____
	_____	_____
	_____	_____
	_____	_____
COATS - 2		
1 rain or trench coat	_____	_____
1 overcoat	_____	
ACCESSORIES		
1 scarf	_____	_____
leather briefcase	_____	_____
dark umbrella	_____	_____
watch	_____	_____
leather gloves	_____	_____
1 dozen handkerchiefs	_____	_____

For more details, see the text in this chapter.

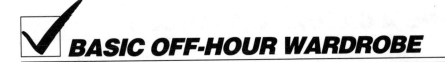

BASIC OFF-HOUR WARDROBE

The following items listed are also based on surveys. The numbers and types of clothing are an average number owned by successful professionals, and for our purposes, are to be considered a minimum requirement for casual wear.

☐ **Jackets:**
- 1 Blazer (solid color)
- 2 Sport jackets (patterned)
- NOTE: If you are in a less-formal industry (real estate, for example) you may wear sport coats and blazers more frequently than suits. Replace 2 suits with extra separates. Example: 3 sport coats, 2 blazers, 7 to 8 pairs slacks.

☐ **Slacks:**
- 4 to 5 pairs of slacks (solid colors)

☐ **Shirts:**
- Three long-sleeve sport shirts
- Two short-sleeve sport shirts
- Four knit sport shirts or polo shirts (Izod, Ralph Lauren, etc.)

☐ **Sweaters:**
- Two solid (crew, v-neck, turtleneck)
- Two patterned

☐ **Neckties:**
- Four "sport" ties (wool, knit, club-style, plaid)

☐ **Belts:**
- Two "sport" belts (fabric and leather combinations, woven and/or colored leathers)

☐ **Socks:**
- Six pairs (solid colors and patterns)

☐ **Shoes:**
- Four pairs (moccasins, loafers, boat shoes, other casuals)

☐ **Coats:**
- Parka/shirt jacket
- Stadium coat
- Windbreaker or battle jacket

BUILDING A CASUAL WARDROBE

Basic Casual Wardrobe	My Actual Wardrobe	Items I Need in My Wardrobe
JACKETS		
1 blazer	_____	_____
2 sport jackets	_____	_____
SLACKS		
4 to 5 pairs	_____	_____
	_____	_____
	_____	_____
SHIRTS		
3 long-sleeve sport shirts	_____	_____
	_____	_____
2 short-sleeve sport shirts	_____	_____
	_____	_____
4 knit polo shirts	_____	_____
	_____	_____
	_____	_____
SWEATERS		
2 solid	_____	_____
2 patterned	_____	_____
	_____	_____

For more details, see the text in this chapter.

BUILDING A CASUAL WARDROBE

Basic Casual Wardrobe	My Actual Wardrobe	Items I Need in My Wardrobe
NECKTIES		
4 sport ties	_____	_____
	_____	_____
BELTS		
2 sport belts: fabric/leather, woven/colors	_____	_____
	_____	_____
SOCKS		
6 pairs: solid, colors, patterns	_____	_____
	_____	_____
SHOES		
4 pairs: moccasins, loafers, boat shoes, etc.	_____	_____
	_____	_____
	_____	_____
COATS		
Parka	_____	_____
Stadium coat	_____	_____
Wind-breaker	_____	_____

For more details, see the text in this chapter.

☐ **Extras for Formal Wear:** These items may be used with the basic corporate/ work wardrobe. They are *must have now* items. Later, a tuxedo and other formal attire can be added. For now, the following will take care of most situations:

- Two all-silk neckties (solid color, dressy paisley or pin-dot)
- Two silk pocket scarves (to complement your neckties, not match them)
- Two French-cuff shirts (white silk or other high-quality fabric)
- One pair of cuff-links (gold or silver, non-ornate)
- One collar bar

Men who have been around and who own extensive wardrobes will also find these lists useful. They may have full closets, but some of the "must have" items may be missing. Men who are just now building a wardrobe for all seasons should concentrate on the specifics; purchase the basics *first*, variety can wait until later.

Putting the Basic Wardrobe Plan into Action

Now that you've got the outlines for a basic wardrobe, the next move is learning how to select and personalize each item. Each of the steps will be discussed in detail later on. For the moment, let's study four primary methods of choosing what's right for you.

In order of importance, the following steps are essential to making a proper choice:

1. Color: While an item of clothing is still on the rack, select the color that's right for you. (The color section will provide a personalized guide.) Don't experiment. "Fashion forward" colors (unusual blends and hues) can be fun, but they aren't serious candidates for your "must have" collection. They can be added later and should be as you learn to express your personality in your dress style for different occasions. Color may not be everything — but it's close. Choose with care.

2. Fabric: We'll get into precise selections of fabric in another chapter, but keep in mind that this category is second in importance, and selections can be made off the rack. What's critical is that fabrics should be natural fibers or blends, not polyesters. Going for the convenience of polyesters is fine for backyard gardening, but pure fibers, such as cotton and wool, say "quality." In recent years, some excellent high-quality blends are available — do look for at least 55 percent natural fiber.

THE BASICS FOR MORE FORMAL EVENTS

Basic Formal Wardrobe	My Actual Wardrobe	Items I Need in My Wardrobe
NECKTIES		
2 all-silk: solid, dressy paisley or pin-dot	_____	_____
	_____	_____
SHIRTS		
2 french cuff	_____	_____
	_____	_____
ACCESSORIES		
2 silk pocket squares	_____	_____
	_____	_____
1 pair cuff links, plain, gold or silver	_____	_____
1 collar bar	_____	_____

For more details, see the text in this chapter.

3. Shape: The item to be chosen has to be taken down from the rack to be studied for proper shaping. However, it can remain on the hanger while you're making up your mind about its appropriateness to your body shape. Later we'll discuss body shapes as they relate to the cut of various suits and slacks. The immediate consideration, however, has to do with the basic silhouette you'll get from a particular style of suit or trousers you're buying. Many men overlook this and wind up making expensive and frustrating mistakes.

4. Fit: it's been said that "fit is everything" and there's more than a little truth to this. At this point in the selection process you are actually going to try on the item of clothing. You'd be surprised how many men don't bother with a fitting session; they feel they know the proper measurements and simply instruct the tailor to cut and stretch to a set of verbally communicated specifications. This, too, leads to big mistakes, wasted money, and worse — an ill-fitting article of clothing that may have cost $1,000 or more but that looks like a hand-me-down. *Always insist on a thorough fitting and tailoring job.* If you're rushed, return to the store another time, when you can do it right!

Ready to Roll

Using the basics here, you'll find that you're already well ahead with what you need, how much of it is bottom line, and how to go about making a wise investment in a "must have" wardrobe. This all may seem too simplistic, but, in fact, these are the rudiments; they are fundamental and you need to know them in detail. Their proper use is invaluable.

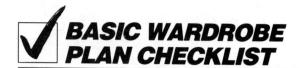

BASIC WARDROBE PLAN CHECKLIST

☐ **Use the lists in Chapter One** *to outline the bottom-line articles* of clothing you'll need at work, during leisure times, and when the occasion demands a more formal look.

☐ **Don't short yourself.** You'll need at least three suits for the office (and at least two others when you can afford them) and a minimal amount of jackets and slacks for casual wear. All those ties and shirts are necessary, too. After all, you'll want a clean shirt every day, and there has to be a spare when the others are at the laundry. Better too many than too few of anything when it comes to looking your best.

☐ **The formalizing accessories are critical.** To be appropriate for such occasions, you need to dress at least one cut above your best office attire. At some point you'll probably need a tuxedo and all the trimmings; but, in the meantime, the list of accessories will give you just enough to get by in reasonable style. They provide a means of looking "dressy" without overdoing it. Mixing and matching will achieve great results.

☐ **Selecting your clothing in specific order: color, shape, fabric, fit.** This is the easiest and most logical way to make your picks. Remember the absolute importance of proper fit, and take your time getting it right. The right color, fabric, and shape can be utterly destroyed by bad tailoring.

☐ **Go for high quality — the very best you can afford.** Remember that your wardrobe is an investment in your own future. And, like any wise investment, it will pay substantial rewards.

CHAPTER TWO

●●

BASIC LOOKS

Why Do I Need All These Clothes?

Lifestyles have changed tremendously in the past 20 years, and men are routinely faced with the demand to adjust their appearance to fit any number of situations.

Gone are the days when it was enough to own a few good suits and a smattering of leisure items. The nuclear age has geometrically multiplied opportunities, and, at the same time, has placed men in the position of being quick-change artists. Today's super mobility requires an office wardrobe, a travel wardrobe, a line of sporting outfits, formal wear, even special items for a backyard barbeque. Some men resent these wardrobe demands and steadfastly refuse to give in to the changing patterns of the life in the 1980s; proudly they tell their colleagues how much money they're saving by sticking to a dress code written in a previous generation. That's fine up to a point. But these stoical "refuseniks" pay a big price in the long run. Fairly or otherwise, their mobility is limited; their appearance says they are either inflexible or unaware (or both!) of the demands of modern life, and the unwritten laws of the times work forcefully against them. Quite simply, their opportunities become frozen.

Does this mean that you'll only go as far as the number of outfits hanging in your closet will allow? Well, maybe not. Perhaps you can make it to the top on sheer guts, brains, and force of will. Like the late Howard Hughes, it may be possible to be a millionaire with a single suit, a shirt, and one tie, and a pair of well-used sneakers. Maybe. But why, in today's ultra-competitive environment, would anyone deliberately limit their options? Let's be realistic. If your wardrobe isn't as varied and expansive as the opportunities around you, you're taking more of a risk than you should reasonably be asked to assume. You certainly want diversity in your investment portfolio and the same prudent, sensible approach needs to be at work in your wardrobe.

Three Basic Male "Looks"

Between Hollywood, television, fiction writers, and a monolithic menswear industry, a misconception has arisen that men are neatly split into one of three types. Conveniently, each so-called type is said to bear (presumably for life) one of three different "looks." These are:

1. The rugged outdoor type: This is the man with craggy features, weathered skin, strong hands, piercing eagle-like eyes, and the physique of a body builder. When it comes to dress, he's pictured in a lumberjack outfit or a thick sheepskin coat and steel-toed boots.

2. The romantic type: This image ranges from a facsimile of Fred Astaire in top hat and tails, to the racey character of Sonny Crockett, the vice cop made famous by Don Johnson of T.V.'s "Miami Vice." The operative word for these "romantics" is "dandy." They're fast on their feet, quick on the draw, and utterly devastating when it comes to the ladies.

3. The successful type: In this scenario we find the captains of the industry such as Chrysler Chairman Lee Iacocca, or billionaires such as philanthropist Armand Hammer. These types are pictured in $3,000 three-piece suits, priceless hand-painted silk neckties, and wing-tip shoes custom-made on Saville Row of the finest leathers.

These images are problematical and confusing, as most cliches tend to be. They are also misleading. The rugged outdoorsman, the romantic, and the successful magnate are one-dimensional cutouts, great if you're dealing in fiction but absurd when it comes to understanding what men are all about. Other cutouts can be added to the list, but these would compound the misunderstanding.

Closer to reality is the fact that most men cross all lines, real and imaginary. Even women, who often fall into the habit of typing males as if they could be slotted into one of three pigeon holes, are beginning to realize that real people are as diverse as the situations they find themselves in. Yes, there are types; but more often than not they are transformed continually by mood and circumstances. Men, like everything else in nature, have only one constant: change!

Looks for All Occasions

In the real world men need different looks for differing situations. While they may be more comfortable in certain specific outfits that more-or-less correspond to the cliched "types," there are times and places that demand different looks.

Instead of stereotyping men, it's far more practical to define styles of dress that are appropriate for situations that arise constantly in the course of modern living.

Fashion designers have capitalized on this idea, providing endless options, with choices of colors, patterns, designs. Men, though enjoying a certain amount of liberation in the choices of style, are often faced with an overabundance of choices that can be more than slightly bewildering. It is therefore even more important to understand the basics within which to work to select an *appropriate* and *credible* wardrobe that fits any occasion.

Real Life Looks that Work

The following looks, or wardrobe designs, correspond to the basic wardrobe plans discussed in Chapter One. Each category describes in a practical, no-nonsense way the various looks you'll need to be your best in most situations. The primary logic behind each is "The Big A" — *Appropriateness.*

Classic Look: Every man needs a classic look — which translates simply as a conservative business suit. The corporate male needs at least five conservative suits. And he needs them for a variety of settings: board meetings, interviews, speaking engagements, political meetings. For these occasions, only the classic look is appropriate. Some industries allow for more high fashion details but conservatism is the norm.

This classic outfit must physically complement the wearer, it must be of good quality and construction, and importantly, the style needs to be *current.*

A note on currency before I go on:

Current doesn't mean "fashion-forward" or faddish. A suit of current design is one that isn't obviously outdated. Do you recall the suits of the rebellious Flower Power Sixties? They had very wide lapels (to go with the super-wide neckties of the era) and the trousers were often bell bottoms. Wearing such a suit today, regardless of its quality, says something quite unflattering about your sense of taste and appropriateness. It says, in the vernacular of the Sixties, that you're "out of it, man!" Wearing a modern design says you're part of today's scene, aware of the here and now. That's the critical message of current style, and it shouldn't be taken lightly.

There are times when the appropriateness of a suit, often its color, is of utmost importance. I'll describe what types of suits, colors, and fabrics are correct and complementary for each of you later on.

Natural Look: Natural can be interchanged with "casual." For a day off, a picnic, a vacation, or almost any leisure situation, this is the way to go.

Natural or casual attire can include exercise and athletic wear. These items need to be comfortable and functional and easy to care for. Included are warm-up suits, jogging and tennis outfits, golf clothing, and swimsuits.

Though they represent easy, let-down-and-relax situations, they should be selected for style and quality. Using cut-off jeans for the tennis court may have been okay when you were 16 years old, or can be just fine when you play on your own private court, but they are anything but acceptable for today's well-dressed man.

Again we come to the matter of appropriateness. There are times and places — the golf course, the country club, a game of squash with a business associate — when you need to consider more than comfort. This isn't a license to overdo it with contrived designer outfits, only a caution that the situation requires you to remain aware of the overall image you're hoping to project — your total style.

Other items in the Natural category include slacks, shorts, sweaters, sport shirts, and similar items suitable for travel and general leisure time. They also call for a certain amount of overall image-awareness. For example, it isn't acceptable (or kind to yourself professionally and socially) to wear the trousers from a suit, battered jeans, short bell bottoms of double-knit fabric, or shirts with five-inch collars for casual wear just because you can't bear to part with them. Sure, we all have our share of shaggy dogs in the closet. Perhaps that's where they belong for reasons of sentiment. But don't kid yourself; they don't work in your favor, and wearing them should be consigned to private moments.

More acceptable are good quality blazers and sport coats, well-fitted slacks, shorts, and sport shirts. These should say that you're relaxed, not sloppy. They need to be well cared for and project favorable signals about who and what you are.

There's yet another group — "work clothes." There definitely are times when covering yourself sans image is fine. When you're cutting grass, painting, and doing general chores, utility is the only common sense consideration.

Dressed-up look: Here we're dealing with special occasions, and there are nuances you need to be aware of. For instance, your pin-striped suit and club tie will surely get you by at a wedding or at your favorite restaurant, but wait! Isn't this the same outfit you wore to the office? If so, the image you're projecting is that you just got off and didn't have time to change. Is this the mood you want to project for a special occasion or that special person?

The answer is obvious. Your outfit says "rushed," it may indicate "work-aholic," a duo of signals with possible negative implications.

Dressed up should mean special, a change of mood, a bit of magic. By including articles of clothing listed under this category in Chapter One, you can transform the ordinary into something more elegant and appealing. Though it requires a bit more effort, it's definitely worth it.

Tuxedos and Dinner Jackets: Many men, especially the younger set, will do anything to get out of donning this formalwear. Of course, they'll rent them for a wedding of a good buddy, but they're reluctant to add them as regulars to a wardrobe. With some good reason.

Formal wear is expensive, unless it's purchased second-hand, and it isn't used very often. The investment just doesn't seem to make sense, especially since more necessary articles of clothing consume a fair amount of income to begin with.

This is understandable, particularly for men just beginning their careers. Eventually, as you make gains, the idea of buying a formal line becomes less extraordinary. I've noticed that many men who reach mid- to upper-level management levels have a real need for a black-tie outfit. It comes with the territory.

When you finally do buy formals, make sure you apply the same tailoring controls that go with a pricey business suit. Insist on perfect tailoring, excellent materials, and the best workmanship.

In the meantime, a solid suit, a silk or French cuffed shirt, a silk tie in a solid color or a fine dot, and a silk pocket scarf will do for most dressed-up or semi-formal occasions.

High Fashion: Handle With Care

"High fashion" is a loaded phrase. Even in the industry that produces it there's constant debate about what it actually implies. High fashion was originally designed for the female market and began easing into the men's area after World War II. Women are used to it; men have been far more reluctant. Over the past two decades, men have shown a bit more tolerance for, and acceptance of, the radical lines that characterize this genre. Still, only a tiny sliver of the total high fashion output is directed at men.

The controversial nature of high fashion should serve as a caution to all — especially men — who flirt with the possibility of including such items in a wardrobe.

Despite the controversy, high fashion comes down to a rather simple definition: it is nothing more than an exaggeration of line, scale, or detail.

Another characteristic is its limited lifetime. Every year (or less) high fashion changes dramatically; if it didn't, it wouldn't live up to its reputation as a fast-paced indicator of the times. Good fashion (less exaggerated) has a 3 to 5 year slowly moving cycle — changes appear slowly and gradually.

Some style experts insist that high fashion is a woman's prerogative and that men should keep a safe distance from it. They believe it's okay for women to experiment, to add a trace of mystery to their wardrobes, because women, they claim, are expected to be slightly frivolous in these matters. Men, on the other hand, are expected to take a more sober approach; they should be neither mysterious nor frivolous. I don't entirely agree.

High fashion has no place in a corporate environment. I believe this holds for both sexes. In a business setting "fun clothes" that make radical statements do just that — they draw attention, they plead for position, and they get in the way. I never recommend exaggeration in developing your own personal style, especially on the job.

However, every man should be aware of fashion and the direction it's taking. Think of the fashion direction as a mirror image of what is happening in our society. Museum exhibits, movies, even the political environment influence fashion changes and we are all aware of this when purchasing cars, computers, homes, boats, sporting gear. New shapes, colors, sizes, and other details continually confront us. They create interest on many levels, and they remind us that life is changing and will continue to change despite our built-in reluctance to accept it. In this sense, "fashion" in clothing is a kind of social barometer, a precursor of things to come.

Though high fashion is inappropriate in most corporate environments, it does enjoy more acceptance in certain fields. Men in advertising, television, and public relations add high fashion touches all the time. Since these fields are generally considered "creative" (as opposed to the fiduciary role of a bank official or the expected conservatism of an attorney), men working in these areas can practice moderate amounts of fashion flair. It's acceptable and more-or-less expected of "creative types."

But there are times when all men can add fashion touches to their appearance. Dressed-up and casual situations offer such flexibility, as do leisure times.

New colors, designs, fabrics, and patterns, are now available for men and using them in moderation gives you an understanding of fashion direction. They allow you to reach in that direction according to your personality and the appropriateness of the occasion.

Having a Little Fun Won't Hurt

Please don't be entirely put off by fashion. It's fine to try some of the new styles of the season. For example, you may want to wear an unconstructed linen jacket with pushed-up sleeves, while other men will feel more comfortable with a more conservative linen blazer. Both would be appropriate for a casual cocktail party at poolside. They would be current and fashionable, and would reflect an individual's unique personality. The guiding force, once again, is the appropriateness for the occasion. Some men's designers, like Alexander Julian, have added fun and excitement to casual clothes with great color combinations and designs. If you are not ready for a "big move" try a new tie design or sweater pattern.

It's possible to wear some of the wonderful new designs and to do it properly. As you develop your style, you'll feel more comfortable trying out these looks. They'll add spice. So why not be a little daring — at the right time, of course.

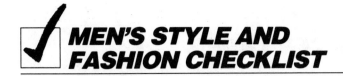

✔ MEN'S STYLE AND FASHION CHECKLIST

☐ **When it comes to dress,** "The Big A" — appropriateness — is as important as what you actually wear. Different occasions demand different looks.

☐ **Avoid "typing" yourself.** Your personality is made up of many moods, many strengths. Make your wardrobe fit your diversity.

☐ **Just about all men need a "classic" look,** a well-made conservative business suit. In a corporate atmosphere you'll need several suits. These should complement you physically, be of good quality, and current in style without being trendy.

☐ **Natural or casual clothes are also critical** to the man on the way up. They should be comfortable and easy to care for. Quality should be high. Don't short yourself by wearing old cut-offs on a tennis court. Even athletic clothing has to be right for your overall image.

☐ **When attending a special occasion,** dress up your look with a French cuff shirt, a solid color silk tie, and pocket scarf. These items take you a cut above your corporate image.

☐ **Think of your wardrobe purchases as an investment.** When buying, go for quality, classic designs, flexibility, durability, comfort, and a flattering fit. They pay big rewards.

☐ **Get rid of outdated clothes.** It's important to be in style — not ahead or behind the curve. Being fashionable doesn't mean "high fashion" or trendy. Current is where you want to be.

☐ **"High fashion"** — exaggerations in line, detail, or scale — isn't a no man's land. You can have fun with these additions to your wardrobe as long as you know exactly when and where to try them out.

☐ **It's important to be aware of fashion trends,** just as you're aware of trends in other areas of your life. To avoid them entirely may be playing too safe, and playing it too safe conveys a stuffy image.

☐ **The purchase of a tuxedo** or a dinner jacket can wait until you've put together a well-rounded wardrobe to fit most everyday demands. Eventually, however, you'll want to own your own formals. Insist on the highest quality materials and workmanship. Few items of clothing miss the mark so completely as bargain-basement formals. It's probably better to buy a top quality second-hand outfit than a cut-rate new one.

CHAPTER THREE

BODY LINES

The Shape You're In

This chapter is aimed at sizing up your specific body shape and size. Used properly, it's the next best thing to a custom tailor.

Before you're through, you'll understand the styles that suit you best, that flatter you, and give you an extra edge in appearance. You'll also learn how the shape of your face dictates the most complementary hairstyle, eyeglasses, shirts, and neckties.

None of this is guesswork or opinion. As promised earlier, the advice offered in based on actual test cases. My company, Accolade, Inc., and its worldwide network of Always In Style consultants have worked with thousands of men and women. The formulas we've developed eliminate, as much as possible, the purely subjective variables that sometimes make suiting-up a hit-or-miss proposition. What you'll find in the following pages is designed to put your particular body and face into the most flattering and (equally important) comfortable outfits.

Fashion in Perspective

Before we go on, a few vital notes on that curious word, "fashion," compared with style.

Fashion is a concept that causes a great deal of confusion for many men. That's understandable. After all, women, who spend a lot more of their time tracking fashion, still make costly errors because of the vagueness of the concept. For some reason it has taken on a kind of intangible quality; it is mercurial, exclusive, even "elitist," and designers have their own special language. No wonder fashion is viewed as being abstract and indefinable.

What exactly is fashion?

Most dictionaries define it as "the way in which something is formed, a configuration." It is also defined as "the prevailing or preferred practice in dress . . . at a given time." It is often a mirror image of what is happening around the world. The changes that continue to happen are reflected in changing styles in clothing as well as other consumer products.

Our matching of body and face shapes is based on the first definition; that is, fashion is a "configuration." We put the right shape with the right outfit.

It's the second definition that appears to cause most of our confusion. A preferred manner of dress at a given time leaves the individual facing a 24-hour-a-day infusion of hype and commercial stimuli. It's a matter of custom or choice; it involves juggling the conflicting opinions of everyone around you, not the least of which are the commercial fashion czars who compete for your disposable income and a commanding market share.

The end result of this assault on the senses is that many men become "fashion victims." Attempting to be stylish, they wind up being trendy or faddish. Their wardrobes become eclectic. And none of this comes cheaply.

The Difference Between Fashion and Style

Your individual style is *you* — who you are, your talents, your looks, your special way of doing things. Your style is forever, and it doesn't change with fashion. It is important to identify your personal style and update it by being aware of the fashion direction.

It is your style that is behind the clothes you select. By defining your body shape as a physically inherent style, it becomes a logical or scientific exercise to pick items that complement that style.

Your clothing has to be personal — a direct and natural extension of you. When you're in a suit that enhances your physical characteristics, it's you and not the suit that gets the most (and best!) attention.

For clothes to complement you physically, they need to be right for your body, fit perfectly, and accent your basic coloring. Once you understand your particular characteristics, you'll make the right choices. Then it's a matter of keeping up with the changes — fashion — and keeping them in line with your special style.

If your clothing is to be a natural extension of you, there needs to be a balance, a harmony, between line, scale, and color. The line of your clothing is the silhouette of the outfit on your body. The patterns, fabrics, and textures need to harmonize in direct proportion to this line.

The scale — size — should be in proportion to the size of your body. As for color, whatever you wear should blend with your natural skintones, hair, and eyes.

In the following section, we'll move step-by-step through line, scale, and color. You'll learn how to analyze yourself and determine exactly what to look for when you go shopping. With this clear-cut information in hand you can overcome bewildering fashion hype and never again become a "fashion victim."

The Geometry of Face Shapes

Before determining your body shape, it's important to accurately determine the shape of your face — the first thing that we see when we look directly at someone. It is part of the total shape of the person and, therefore, the first step in analyzing your body shape. It also allows you to make flattering choices in hairstyles, shirts, and eyeglass frames. As usual, the idea is to eliminate hit-or-miss perceptions about what's best for you.

Forget ideals. It's really pointless, for instance, to follow the advice of those who insist that hairstyles and glasses should somehow *change* your face. It

IDENTIFYING YOUR FACE SHAPE

Sharp-Straight

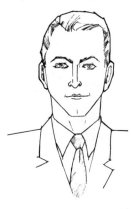

The Sharp-Straight face shape is made up of straight lines. Features such as: nose, jawline, cheekbones and chin are chiseled and very angular. Lips are often thin. A single sharp feature does not constitute a Sharp-Straight face. It is the overall impression of angularity that matters.

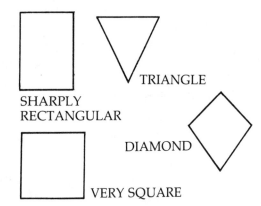

SHARPLY RECTANGULAR

TRIANGLE

DIAMOND

VERY SQUARE

Straight

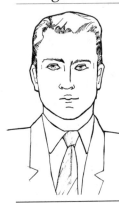

A Straight face shape is made up of straight lines. Features; nose, jawline and chin can be straight, rectangular or square. Lips are neither thin nor very full. A single straight line feature does not constitute a Straight face. It is the overall impression of straightness that matters.

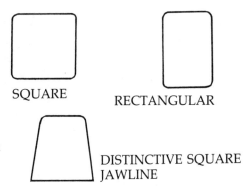

SQUARE

RECTANGULAR

DISTINCTIVE SQUARE JAWLINE

Contoured

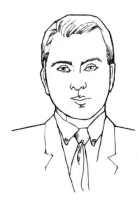

The Contoured face shape is made up of curved lines. Features; nose, jawline, cheeks and chin are rounded. Lips are often full. There are no well defined angles. A single rounded feature does not constitute a Contoured face. It is the overall impression of curved lines that matters.

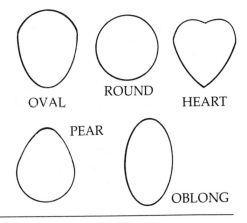

OVAL

ROUND

HEART

PEAR

OBLONG

WHERE IS YOUR FACE'S SHAPE ON THE CONTINUUM?

☐ Sharp nose
☐ Angular, well defined jaw
☐ Thin lips
☐ Strong cheekbones
☐ Pointed chin
☐ Well defined angles

☐ Square nose
☐ Square jaw
☐ Average size lips
☐ Defined cheekbones
☐ Square chin
☐ Angles

☐ Rounded nose
☐ Rounded, softly definited jaw
☐ Full, rounded lips
☐ Cheekbones not prominent
☐ No prominent chin
☐ Absence of angles

VERY SHARP FEATURES & FACE SHAPE	SHARP	STRAIGHT FEATURES & FACE SHAPE	CONTOUR	VERY CONTOURED FEATURES & FACE SHAPE

You may not be able to exactly describe your face as one of the *Successful Style* prototypes. But to choose your best collar styles and patterns for ties you need to know which of the three is the closest to your face shape—or where you are on the continuum.

doesn't work that way. After all, your face shape is determined by DNA. Bone structure and the arrangement of muscle and flesh don't give way to cosmetic dabbling. It's certainly possible to correct minor problems with hairstyles and beards, a subject to be discussed in detail later on. But the bottom line is fairly simple: You aren't going to fool Mother Nature! Your face is an immutable part of who you are. Learn to recognize its basic shape and learn how to make the most of it.

The standard face shapes are oval, pear, heart, round, rectangle, triangle, square — combinations of these naturally exist. For simplicity we will consider those described in the charts in this chapter.

Notice that the seven face shapes can be grouped into two categories:

- Shapes composed of straight lines: square, rectangle, diamond, triangle.

- Shapes composed primarily of curved lines: oval, round, oblong, pear, heart.

Naturally there are faces that are made up of straight and curved lines. Rather than deciphering all the combinations, simply determine if your face is generally straight-lined or contoured.

You'll notice that face and body shapes can be drawn with various lines and geometric figures. We're going to combine face and body lines to determine the overall impression or image you project from head to toe.

Body Shapes

Tall, short, thin, fat, muscular, broad — these are among the many words used to describe the masculine physique. Unfortunately, the terms are vague and misleading; there's no specific definition for any of them. This vagueness is one of the reasons men make inaccurate clothing selections.

The confusion is often compounded by menswear retailers. Many clothing stores segment their lines under these and other hopelessly generalized terms. No wonder there are so many "white elephants" in the closet!

Implicit in these terms is the notion of an "ideal" body shape. That's another mistake. There is no ideal. We're all individuals and no one shape or size is more or less better than any other.

The secret of making the right choice in clothing depends on *accurately* defining your specific body shape. With a good working definition in-hand, you can select items that emphasize your positive characteristics and hide the minor flaws. This is an important step in developing a personal style.

The charts in this chapter outline just about every variation in men's body lines. See where you fit in the *Sharp-straight*, *Straight*, and *Contoured* categories.

Using the Universal Body Shape Concept

Fortunately, men aren't blessed (or cursed, depending on your point of view) with the seemingly endless variety of body shapes that we find among females. The three shapes shown in the chart — sharp-straight, straight, and contoured — describe most men, regardless of their height or weight. Let's examine the three categories in more detail.

Sharp-straight: These men are quite angular. They have flared and squared shoulders, tapered hips, and erect posture. No matter how heavy or thin they may be, their shoulder expanse, ribcage, and hip structure project a distinctive triangular shape. Many sharp-straight men also have facial features to match: lots of straight lines and "chiseled" features. The total image projected is one of angularity.

Study the figure at right and notice the geometric overlay on page 43. This is the classic sharp-straight physique.

Straight: Moving along the continuum, the body lines are less severe. In the straight male figure the shoulders may still be square, but there's less difference between shoulder or chest span and the width of the hips.

A rectangular or square face, or a square jaw line, is typical of this the straight body type. Facial features and angles tend to be less extreme than those of the sharp-straight type.

Notice the straight body shape at right and see how it reveals gradual movement from the sharp-straight to the straight. Notice the change in the geometric overlays on page 47.

Contoured: This third type may still be described as more-or-less rectangular. However, the shoulders are sloping and muscle and flesh are arranged in such a way that the edges appear somewhat rounded.

The contoured body type has facial features that are more rounded; typical are the pear, heart, oval, and circular features. Neck widths are often larger, projecting a "stocky" appearance. This has nothing to do with actual body weight. It's a function of the way muscle and flesh are arranged around a specific bone structure. Notice the geometric overlays on page 45.

CONSIDER THREE
IDENTIFIABLE BODY SHAPES

Sharp-Straight	*Straight*	*Contoured*

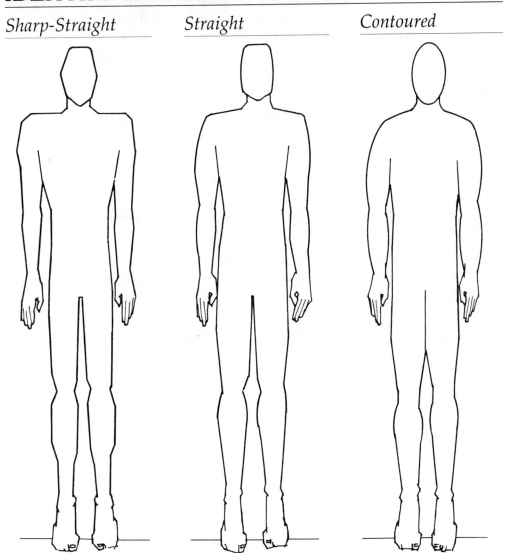

Tall, short, thin, fat, muscular, stocky—these are among the many words used to describe the masculine physique. The terms are vague and misleading: there is no specific definition in any of them.

The secret to making the right choice in clothing depends on accurately defining your specific body shape.

This chart shows three distinct categories: Sharp-Straight, Straight, and Contoured.

Where do you fit in? Look at the charts on the following pages to learn more about which category best describes you.

Sharp-straight Men

Sharp-straight bodied men have broad shoulders and narrow hips. They will have more than a 7″ drop between chest and waist size. Often they're described in romantic language. "Dashing" is a much-used word for sharp-straight types.

Their facial features include chiseled lines with a clean, broad jaw. Angular, lean, and often muscled, they march across the movie and TV screens of the world and are idealized by both sexes.

When sharp-straight men put on too much weight, they develop pot bellies. Generally they don't blimp out, as many contoured men do. It's hard to say if this is a blessing or less, but is a fact of male anatomy.

The celebrated sharp-straight men in our lives include Sylvester Stallone, the "Italian Stallion" of the *Rocky* epics. Stallone is only five-feet seven-inches tall, but his workout routines make him look bigger. If he ever allows himself to get out of shape, he might well go the direction of Oliver Hardy.

Actor Pierce Brosnan, and Christopher Reeve of *Superman* fame also fit the sharp-straight image. Other similarly proportioned matinee idols are the suntanned George Hamilton and Gregory Hines, the fabulous tap dancer.

Two other examples are John Kennedy, Jr., and the outspoken music man, Frank Zappa, formerly of the "Flower Child" generation.

WHAT IS YOUR BODY SHAPE?

Body Type: Sharp-Straight

Does your body resemble the Sharp-Straight man shown at right?

There are three body types for you to look at in this chapter: Sharp-Straight, Straight and Contoured.

Sharp-Straight men are quite angular. They have flaired and squared shoulders, tapered hips, and erect posture, no matter how heavy or thin they may be. Their shoulder expanse, rib cage, and hip structure projects a distinctive triangular shape. Many Sharp-Straight men also have facial features to match: lots of straight lines and "chiseled" features. The total image projected is one of angularity.

The diamonds and triangles drawn over the body are geometric shapes characteristic of this body type.

Face Shape: Square, Diamond, Inverted triangle

Body Shape: Triangular, Exaggerated shoulders

Overall Impression: Angularity, Sharp straight lines

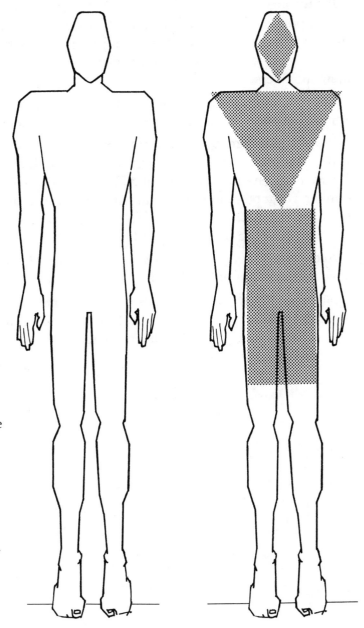

Look elsewhere in this chapter for a side by side comparison of the three body types.

The Contoured Man

"Contoured" men may have rounded features. They aren't angular and they have almost none of the Brutus "lean and hungry look."

It's incorrect to lump contoured men into the overweight category, though extra pounds surely weigh in that direction. The primary guideline is that contoured men have generally round faces and soft features. Their bodies typically present the same (or close to it) measurements from hips to their shoulders.

They have ample proportions, and when they put on too much weight they appear bulky, overly round, especially in the mid-section.

Prototypical contoured men are comedians Randy Quads, Dom DeLouise and writer/producer Rob Reiner (you may recall him as "Meathead" in *All In The Family*). The male lead in that TV show, Carroll O'Connor, a/k/a Archie Bunker, is a good example of what happens when a contoured man plumps up. Johnny Carson, though thin, has an oval face with few if any angles and fits into the chart near the contoured position.

Actor Jeff Bridges is another contoured man. He isn't plump, but he does have soft, non-angular features.

Singer/composer Paul Simon is contoured. He's actually quite slender, but his features are smooth. The quintessential contoured man was the late great Louis Armstrong. It would be hard to find any sharp edges anywhere on "Satchmo."

WHAT IS YOUR BODY SHAPE?

Body Type: Contoured

Does your body resemble the Contoured man shown at right?

There are three body types for you to look at in this chapter: Sharp-Straight, Straight and Contoured.

Contoured men can be described as more-or-less rectangular. The shoulders are sloping and muscle and flesh are arranged in such a way that the edges appear somewhat rounded.

The Contoured body type has facial features that are more rounded; typical are the pear, heart, oval, and circular features. Neck widths are often larger, projecting a "stocky" appearance. This has nothing to do with actual body weight. It's a function of the way muscle and flesh are arranged around a specific bone structure.

The ovals and softened rectangles drawn over the body are geometric shapes characteristic of this body type.

Face Shape: Oval, Round, Oblong

Body Shape: Rectangular (softened edges), Ellipse

Overall Impression: Elliptical, Contoured lines

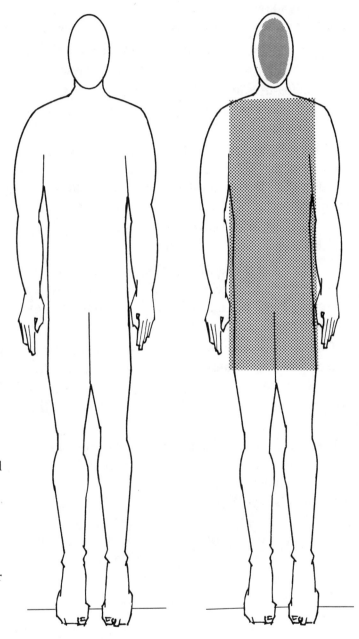

Look elsewhere in this chapter for a side by side comparison of the three body types.

In Between: The Straight Man

Straight-bodied men are characterized by hips and shoulders that are approximately the same. They will have a 6″ or less drop in chest and waist size. The body may be boxy or rectangular, and sometimes it's difficult to tell them apart from either contoured or sharp-straight physiques.

There's an old Gaelic description that seems perfect for straight men: "The broad backs of the Irish . . ." Straight up and down!

Facial features are neither round nor angular but appear more straight. When they put on extra pounds they get broader so that it's hard to tell the muscle from the flab.

Sidney Poitier is a straight type, as is the boxy Robert Mitchum. Others include actor Robert Redford, Hawaiian "PI" Tom Selleck, and talk-show dynamo Phil Donahue. Both funny men Bill Cosby and David Letterman also fit into this slot.

If you can't tell if you're a straight or a sharp-straight, chances are you're the former.

See if you fit these charts. Notice the continuum. Everyone is an individual and can find a unique position on the graph, but we are talking about a general "direction" and not trying to categorize inadvertently. Consider if you are more sharp or more contoured.

The best way to check your body shape is to stand in front of a full-length mirror wearing underwear, a bathing suit, or close-fitting sportswear. Study the silhouette or exterior line of the body, the slope of your shoulders, the "drop" between your chest and waist. Also study your face shape to see how it works with your body line.

Everyone can find his body shape somewhere on the chart. Your body line will remain consistent. Over the years, the flesh will shift somewhat, often with the addition of some extra pounds. But this won't affect your bone structure; it will only change the range or position of your body on the chart. The sharp-straight man may move toward straight, and the straight-lined man may shift somewhat toward a contoured shape. However, it's unlikely that you'll experience a radical movement from one category to another.

WHAT IS YOUR BODY SHAPE?

Body Type: Straight

Does your body resemble the Straight man shown at right?

There are three body types for you to look at in this chapter: Sharp-Straight, Straight and Contoured.

Straight men have body lines that are less severe. The straight man's shoulders may be square, but there's less difference between shoulder or chest span and the width of the hips.

A rectangular or square face, or a square jaw line, is typical of this the Straight body type. Facial features and angles tend to be less extreme than those of the Sharp-Straight type.

The squares and rectangles drawn over the body are geometric shapes characteristic of this body type.

Face Shape: Square, Rectangular, Square jaw

Body Shape: Rectangular, Square

Overall Impression: Rectangular, Straight lines

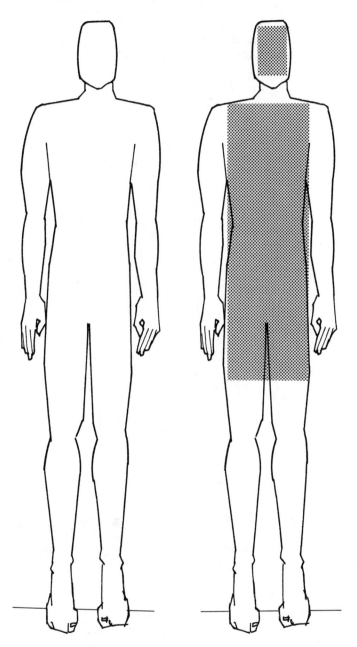

Look elsewhere in this chapter for a side by side comparison of the three body types.

WHERE DO YOU FIT ON THE CONTINUUM?

Everyone has a unique body shape. You may not fit perfectly into one of the three *Successful Style* body shape categories. Determine where you fit on the continuum. Are you more sharp than contoured?

Do you have an angular face or a round one?

Do you have wide shoulders and "no" hips, or are you more straight up and down?

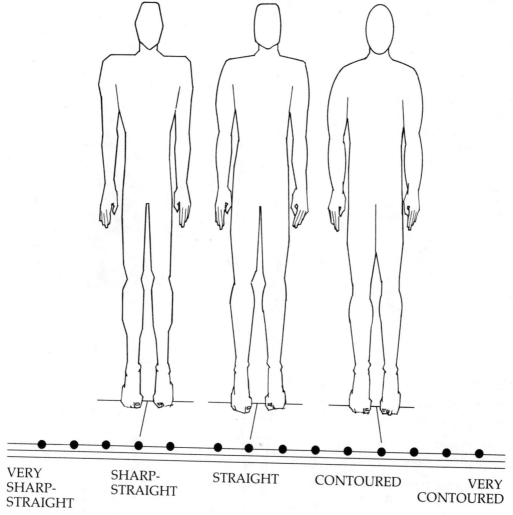

VERY
SHARP-
STRAIGHT
    SHARP-
    STRAIGHT
    STRAIGHT
    CONTOURED
    VERY
    CONTOURED

By understanding your body shape, you will be able to identify exactly which clothes will make you look your absolute best.

Read the text for examples of men who exemplify these body shapes. Remember that it is a continuum. What's important to know is if you are basically Sharp-Straight, Straight or Contoured.

    BODY LINES

Matching Clothing and Body Lines

Now that you've determined your body line, you're ready to select clothing that will be a natural extension of your particular geometry. Using this system, your clothing will take on a custom-tailored look.

There are two types of lines, or details, to consider: *silhouette lines* and *detail lines*.

Silhouette lines: This is the *exterior outline* of a suit — its shape.

Detail lines: These include styling touches such as the shape of pocket flaps, top stitching, amount of shoulder padding, type of fabric and its design.

Silhouette Lines

In studying the shape (silhouette) of a suit, it may be helpful to recall a principle of geometry that defines a line as an infinite number of points moving in a direction. The direction is either straight or curved. A shape can be formed with straight lines and angles, curved lines, or a combination. With this as a reference point, let's look at different suit shapes and match them with the various body line.

Brooks Brothers Style: Three-button, soft shoulder, little waist emphasis.

Modified ("Updated") American: Straight lines, square shoulders, indented waist.

European Style: Peaked lapels, square shoulders, waist emphasis, high cut armhole.

Notice how the suit shapes coordinate with the body lines.

Following descriptions of the three types of suits will help you match-up and coordinate the lines.

Brooks Brothers, "Ivy League," "Sack":
- Little or no padding in shoulders.
- Little or no shaping at the waist.
- Deep-cut armholes.
- Single-breasted; typically center venter.
- Plain front trousers; trouser waist drop usually five inches from coat size.
- Three- to three-and-a-half inch width lapels.
- Three-button or high closure jacket.
- May have cuffed trouser.

The general silhouette of this type of suit has been softened to mold more easily around the body with a less angular projection.

Updated American (Modified-European):
- Moderate waist shaping.
- Generally single-breasted; may be double-breasted.
- Single- or double-vented jacket.
- Shaped shoulder with padding.
- Armholes cut higher; notched lapels; closes a little lower on chest. Notch may be dropped or have wide split.
- Can have pleated or plain front trousers.
- Trouser waist is smaller, often a six- to seven-inch drop from jacket size.

This suit projects a straight line, but there is no extreme exaggeration of the line.

European Cut:
- Snugly fitted waist with tapered hips; often no belt loops; button sewn in for braces.
- Double-breasted; occasionally single-breasted.
- Usually side-vented or non-vented jacket.
- Trouser drop seven inches or more.
- Square shoulders, heavily padded.
- High-cut armholes.
- Wider lapels, usually peaked, may have higher notch.
- Low button closure on jacket.
- Trousers often pleated, with or without cuffs.
- Occasional cuff on jacket sleeve.
- Low-rise trousers.
- Pant leg fuller in the seat.

The European cut projects the sharpest lines and angles necessary to, and complementary of, a very angular body shape. European cut does not mean "made in Europe" but refers to the shape.

Summing Up Suit and Body Lines

All of the silhouettes shown here project a certain feel, a line, and style. The Brooks Brothers, or sack suit, gives a soft effect; there are no sharp or exaggerated lines. It's feel is generally relaxed. There's a bit of contouring at the shoulders, waist, and hips. This is an easy wearing suit for the contoured man.

The European silhouette is just the opposite. It's very straight, with sharp angles, and exaggerated square shoulders. The straight line does not have to be

YOU WILL FIND MORE THAN JUST THREE KINDS OF SUITS

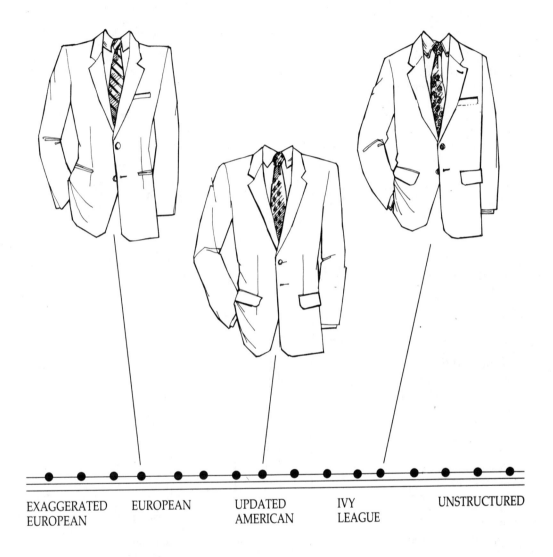

EXAGGERATED   EUROPEAN   UPDATED   IVY   UNSTRUCTURED
EUROPEAN   AMERICAN   LEAGUE

You will find suits that are perfect examples of the three basic styles of suits defined in *Successful Style:* European, Updated American and Ivy League. Variations of these types are available.

Train your eye to identify the dominant character of an individual suit while it is still on the hanger. Understanding its shape and your own will tell you how it is going to fit before you try it on.

CHOOSING YOUR IDEAL CUT OF SUIT

The Sharp-Straight body & the European-cut suit

If you have a Sharp-Straight body, the European cut suit will look like a natural extension of your physique. It is very straight, sharply angled, and has exaggerated shoulders.

Men who are conservative by nature, or who work in conservative companies, will want to avoid highly stylized versions of the European cut.

Selecting a crisp pattern or fabric will make the Updated American straighter and provide a more conservative option.

But in every case, the suit's line must be coordinated with the shape of your body. It's this coordination that gives you the most natural look.

SHOULDER: Square shoulders, padded.

ARMHOLES: High-cut.

LAPELS: Exaggerated lapels, often peaked, may have higher notch.

WAIST: Emphasized, double-breasted, occasionally single breasted.

CLOSURE: Low button closure on jacket.

DROP: Trouser drop seven inches or more.

VENTS: Usually side-vented or non-vented jacket.

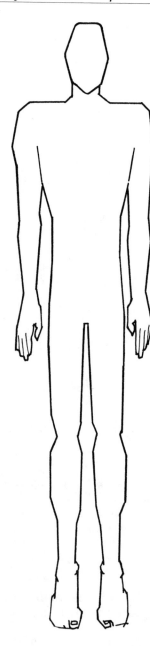

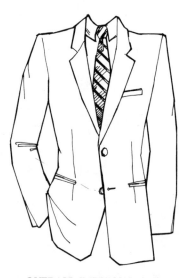

TROUSERS: Loosely fitted waist with tapered hips, often with no belt loops. Buttons sewn in for braces. Often pleated, with or without cuffs. Low-rise. Pant leg fuller in the seat.

OVERALL IMPRESSION: The European cut projects sharp lines and angles. This makes it complementary for a very angular body shape.

European cut does not mean "Made in Europe" but refers to the shape.

HOW TO FIND THIS SUIT: Ask for this suit by name. Tell the salesperson that you are looking for a "European cut".

Then look at the suit on the hanger. Does it have the silhouette and details characteristic of a European cut suit as listed above?

You also want to consider the fabric and color. You will find more information on how fabric influences cut in Chapter four. How to choose the exact color best for you is covered in Chapter seven.

CHOOSING YOUR IDEAL CUT OF SUIT

The Straight body & the Updated American suit

If you have a Straight body, the Updated American cut suit will look like a natural extension of your physique. It is straight, yet does not project an extreme or exaggerated shape.

Selecting a crisp pattern or fabric will make a less straight suit look straighter. Selecting a softer fabric will make a European cut suit less angular, providing a more fashion oriented option.

But in every case, the suit's line must be coordinated with the shape of your body. It's this coordination that gives you the most natural look.

SHOULDER: Shaped shoulder with padding.

ARMHOLES: Standard to high cut armholes.

LAPELS: Notched or peaked lapels. Notch may be dropped or have a wide split.

WAIST: Moderate waist shaping.

CLOSURE: Generally single-breasted, may be double breasted. Closes a little lower on the chest than the Ivy League styles.

DROP: Six- to seven- inch drop from jacket size.

VENTS: Single- or double-vented.

TROUSERS: Pleated or plain front trousers.

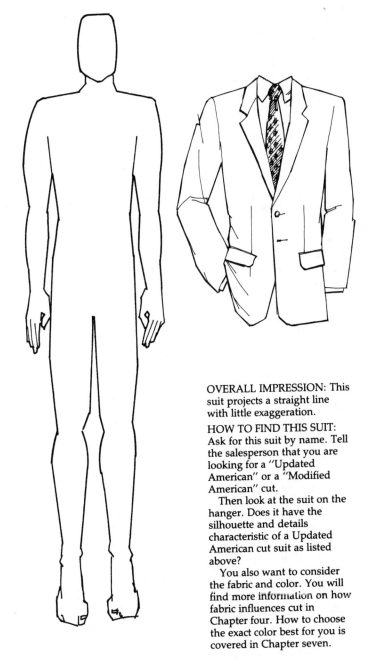

OVERALL IMPRESSION: This suit projects a straight line with little exaggeration.

HOW TO FIND THIS SUIT: Ask for this suit by name. Tell the salesperson that you are looking for a "Updated American" or a "Modified American" cut.

Then look at the suit on the hanger. Does it have the silhouette and details characteristic of a Updated American cut suit as listed above?

You also want to consider the fabric and color. You will find more information on how fabric influences cut in Chapter four. How to choose the exact color best for you is covered in Chapter seven.

CHOOSING YOUR IDEAL CUT OF SUIT

The Contoured body & the Ivy League suit

If you have a Contoured body, the Ivy League suit will look like a natural extension of your physique. It is very gently shaped, without sharp angles or exaggerated shoulders.

Selecting a less crisp pattern or fabric will make the Updated American a less conservative more fashion related option for you.

But in every case, the suit's line must be coordinated with the shape of your body. It's this coordination that gives you the most natural look.

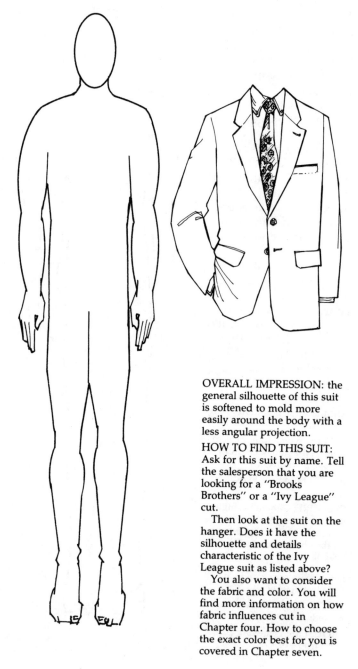

SHOULDER: Little or moderate padding in shoulders.

ARMHOLES: Deep-cut armholes.

LAPELS: Three- to three-and-a-half-inch width lapels, not peaked.

WAIST: Little or no shaping in the waist. Single breasted.

CLOSURE: Three button or high closure jacket is an option.

DROP: Usually five inches from coat size.

VENTS: Typically center vented.

TROUSERS: Plain front trousers. May be cuffed.

OVERALL IMPRESSION: the general silhouette of this suit is softened to mold more easily around the body with a less angular projection.

HOW TO FIND THIS SUIT: Ask for this suit by name. Tell the salesperson that you are looking for a "Brooks Brothers" or a "Ivy League" cut.

Then look at the suit on the hanger. Does it have the silhouette and details characteristic of the Ivy League suit as listed above?

You also want to consider the fabric and color. You will find more information on how fabric influences cut in Chapter four. How to choose the exact color best for you is covered in Chapter seven.

A SUIT EVERYONE CAN WEAR

The Updated American

The Updated American, or a variation of it, is a style of suit that everyone can wear. Fabric makes the difference.

For SHARP-STRAIGHT body lines: A crisper fabric will straighten the line of the Updated American and make the silhouette appropriate for the man whose body line is Sharp-Straight. The option offers a more conservative alternative than the more exaggerated European cut.

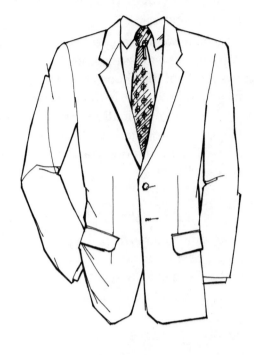

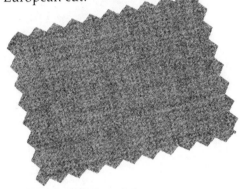

For STRAIGHT body lines: The Updated American is the normal choice for the man with a Straight body line. He should avoid exaggerations of both crispness and softness in the fabric choice.

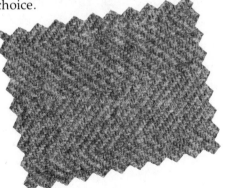

For CONTOURED body lines: When a suit is made of a softer fabric, the silhouette of the Updated American suit will complement the Contoured body shape. This option offers a more fashion oriented alternative.

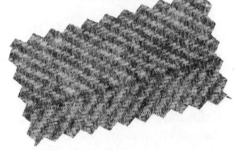

For more detailed information about which fabrics will be the best for you, see Chapter six.

extremely exaggerated. It can simply create a well-defined straight line better suited for an angular body.

To one degree or another these styles reflect different fashion statements. The Brooks (sack) design is more conservative than the highly fitted European lines.

For men who are conservative by nature, or who work in conservative companies, the message is fairly obvious: *avoid the highly styled European cuts*. Of course, any of the shapes can be tuned down or exaggerated even more. Most important, however, is that *the suit line must be coordinated with the shape of your body*. It's this coordination that gives you the most natural look. The modified European or updated American can work for many. The proper selection of fabric will make it more straight or contoured. Fabric selection will be covered in the next chapter.

Face Shapes and Collar Styles

The same geometric principles used to describe suit and body lines apply to face shapes. Later we will see how the various shapes can be used to select a hairstyle and eyeglasses. In this section, we'll look at shirt styles and discover how to achieve the most harmonious look.

Selecting Shirts

There are three basic considerations in picking the right shirt: collar style, fabric, and patterns. Since the collar is the most critical aspect, you need to be aware of the five basic collar types and how they work to complement the different facial contours. Fabric and patterns are included in the chart on clothing lines at the end of the chapter.

Despite the almost limitless selection of shirt collars, the following are basic:

Standard collar: This is the collar worn by most men. It comes in different points, from short to wide, to long and thin. It is typically sold with collar stays. It's appropriate for business, casual, and dressed-up occasions.

Button-down collar: This collar is also quite common. As its name implies, the collar is held down at the points with buttons. It's less dressy than the standard collar and is appropriate for business and casual looks.

Pin collar: The pinned collar gives the shirt a more formal, dressy look. Some collars have holes to accommodate a pin or collar "bar." The pin shouldn't be worn with a wide spread collar or a button-down type.

Tab collar: The tab collar has a similar effect to the pin collar; however, the collar has a small tab of fabric with a snap that is snapped under the tie, drawing the collar in.

Spread collar: The points are short to average and spread far apart. It always projects a dressy look. This shirt goes best with a European style suit and must be worn with a wide knot in the necktie.

Round collar: This shirt can be worn with or without a pin. However, adding the pin gives it a dressy look. This model isn't recommended for business, but it is appropriate for casual and dressed-up occasions.

Whatever your preference in collars, it's critical to pick a style that relates to your face shape and bone structure. The tie pattern can be used to balance a collar shape and relate it to a particular face shape.

A big man with a wide face won't look balanced with a tiny collar. Meanwhile, a collar with long points will overwhelm a small man with an oblong face; it'll make his face look even longer. The general rules is: *the length of the points and the spread of the collar should balance the length and shape of the face.*

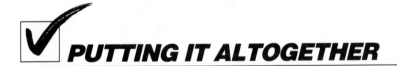

PUTTING IT ALTOGETHER

With only minimal exceptions, the listing of face shapes and collar styles below work quite well for most men. You may find it possible to do a bit of juggling, but the list has been thoroughly tested; it holds up well, and it really works.

☐ **Square face:**
- Standard collar, average to slightly long length, slightly narrow spread.
- Button-down if body is straight and not sharp-straight.
- Pin collar.

☐ **Diamond face:**
- Standard collar, average length, average to slightly wide spread.
- Avoid long points.

THE RIGHT COLLAR STYLE FOR YOUR FACE SHAPE

Sharp-Straight Face Shapes

VERY SQUARE

 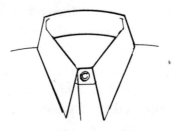 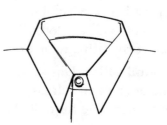

average to slightly long length   narrow spread

TRIANGLE & DIAMOND

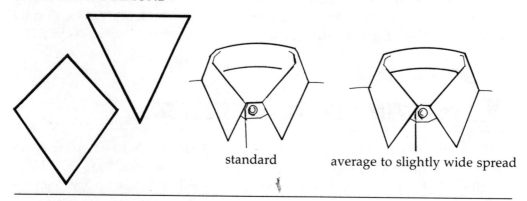

standard   average to slightly wide spread

SHARPLY RECTANGULAR

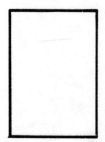 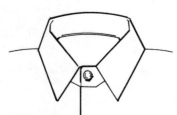 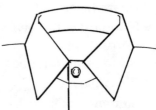

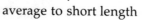

average to short length   average to wide spread

Sharp-Straight Face Shapes

VERY SQUARE

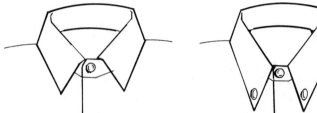

avoid wide spread and short collars   avoid button-down

TRIANGLE & DIAMOND

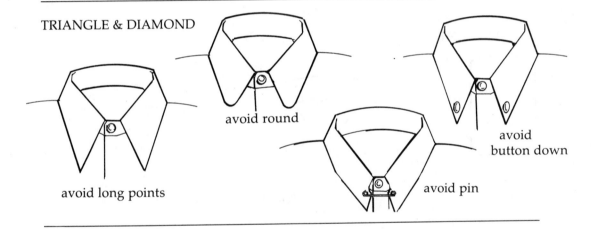

avoid round

avoid long points

avoid pin

avoid
button down

SHARPLY RECTANGULAR

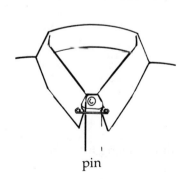

pin

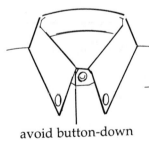

avoid button-down

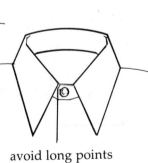

avoid long points

THE RIGHT COLLAR STYLE FOR YOUR FACE SHAPE

Straight Face Shapes

SQUARE

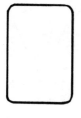

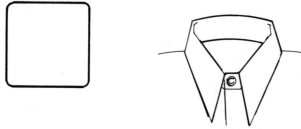

average to slightly long lapels

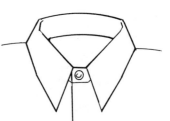

narrow spread

RECTANGULAR

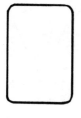

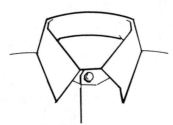

average to short length

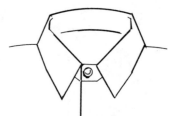

average to wide spread

DISTINCTIVE SQUARE JAWLINE

Select either Square or Rectangular face guidelines depending on length of face.

Straight Face Shapes

SQUARE

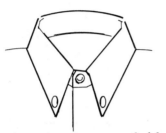

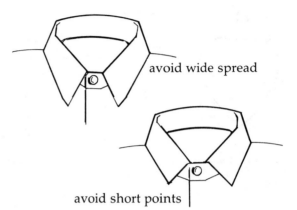

avoid wide spread

button down in crisp, smooth fabric

avoid short points

RECTANGULAR

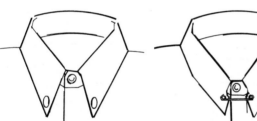

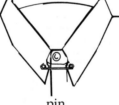

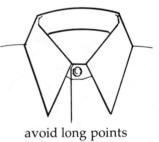

button down in crisp fabric   pin   avoid long points

DISTINCTIVE SQUARE JAWLINE

THE RIGHT COLLAR STYLE FOR YOUR FACE SHAPE

Contoured Face Shapes

HEART

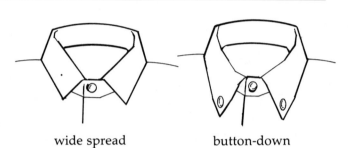

wide spread   button-down

PEAR

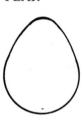

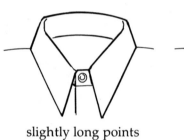
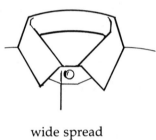

slightly long points   wide spread

OVAL & OBLONG

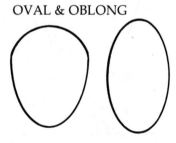

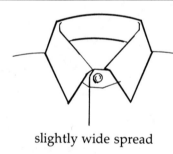
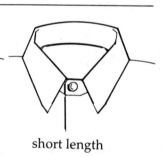

slightly wide spread   short length

ROUND

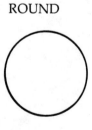

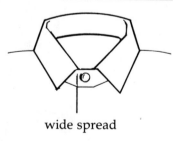
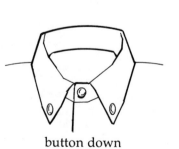

wide spread

button down

Contoured Face Shapes

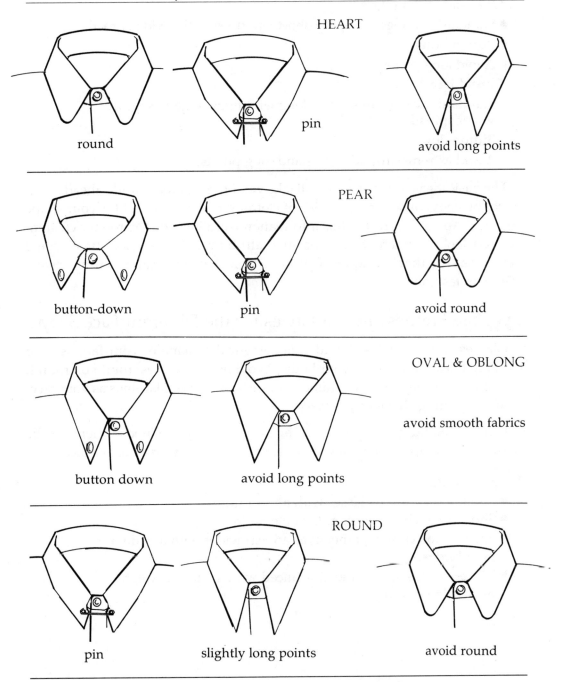

HEART

round

pin

avoid long points

PEAR

button-down

pin

avoid round

OVAL & OBLONG

avoid smooth fabrics

button down

avoid long points

ROUND

pin

slightly long points

avoid round

☐ **Rectangular face:**
- Standard, average to short length, average to wide spread.
- Button-down if body is straight and not sharp-straight.
- Pin collar.

☐ **Oval and Oblong face:**
- Standard, average to slighty short length, slightly wide spread.
- Button-down.
- Avoid long points.

☐ **Round face:**
- Standard, average to slightly long length, average to slightly wider spread.
- Button-down.
- Avoid extremes,round collars and long points.

The basic ideas outlined here will take you orders of magnitude ahead in the tricky business of selecting articles of clothing that are natural for your shape and size. Applied correctly, this information will allow you to project a custom-tailored look and accent your positive attributes. At the same time, you'll develop a style that is uniquely yours — a style that will wear well through any trends in fashion.

Eyeglass Frames and Hairstyles for the Different Face Shape

Glasses and hairstyles should complement the shape of your face as your clothing lines complement your body. Avoid both extremes: round on round, or square on round. Select a frame with the same or similar lines as your face. Avoid repeating shape of your face.

Frames should be the same width as your temple. Choose them a little narrower to compensate for a wide face, or a little wider for a narrow face.

Helpful Hints:
- Long nose, choose glasses with a low bridge.
- Short nose, choose a high, keyhole bridge.
- Small or too close together eyes appear wider with a wide or light bridge.
- Wide-set eyes appear more balanced with a heavier weight, dark-colored bridge.

EYEGLASS FRAMES AND HAIRCUT

Sharp-Straight Face Shapes

VERY SQUARE   Select frames that have some straight lines on top and side. Avoid heavy or wide frames since you are trying to create some length.

   Hairstyle should add width on top and should remain flat on sides. Longer lengths at back will often create the illusion of a longer face.

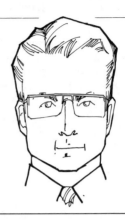

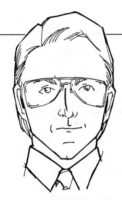

DIAMOND   The diamond face wants to create the illusion of a wider chin line and forehead. Frames with width on the top, straight sides, and weight on the bottom are best. The frame should not have curved edges. Hairstyle should be slightly fuller in back to fill out chin. Sides should be close to face and off-center part used to fill out the forehead. Bangs often work well.

SHARPLY RECTANGULAR   A wide, square frame with a straight bottom is best. The extra width will make the face appear shorter. Select hairstyles that are flat on top. Bangs are especially complementary. Add fullness on sides—avoid long hair at neck.

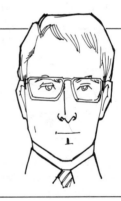

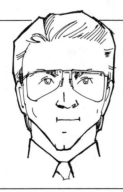

TRIANGLE   Triangular faces have a broad forehead and narrow chin. Frames that are heavier at the bottom are best, filling out chin area. Aviator frames work well if they are straight on the sides.

   Choose hairstyles that are full in the back for weight around chin area. An off-center part will cut the width of the forehead. Use styles that are brushed back or flat of sides.

EYEGLASS FRAMES AND HAIRCUT

Straight Face Shapes

SQUARE   Select frames that have some straight lines on top and side. Avoid heavy or wide frames since you are trying to create some length.

   Hairstyle should add width on top and should remain flat on sides. Longer lengths at back will often create the illusion of a longer face.

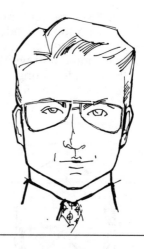

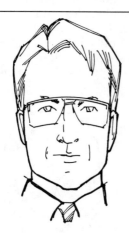

RECTANGULAR   A wide, square frame with a straight bottom is best. The extra width will make the face appear shorter.

   Select hairstyles that are flat on top. Bangs are especially complementary. Add fullness on sides— avoid long hair at neck.

DISTINCTIVE SQUARE JAWLINE   Select frames that have some straight lines on top and sides. Avoid heavy or wide frames since you are trying to create some length.

   Hairstyles should add width on top and should remain flat on sides. Longer lengths at back will often create the illusion of a longer face.

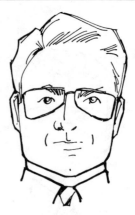

EYEGLASS FRAMES AND HAIRCUT

Contoured Face Shapes

OVAL   An oval face can wear any frame that is not extreme. Avoid harsh angles.

Any current hairstyle works well if it is appropriate for your lifestyle and personality.

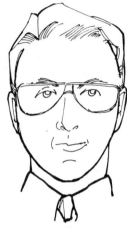

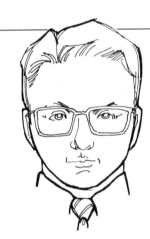

ROUND   Avoid round glasses or curved sides, which will emphasize roundness. Select a shape that has the edges "knocked-off" so that a contoured shape is obvious without creating a circle. A straight line across the top will create balance.

Select hairstyles with width on top and flat on sides. An off-center part will cut the forehead giving a more slender look. Layered looks add softness.

OBLONG   Choose slightly wide, square frames with rounded sides. Extra width shortens face.

A hairstyle with the same fullness on side and flatness on top works for the oblong face as it does for the rectangular. A softer layered cut complements the contoured lines.

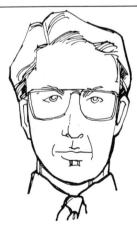

EYEGLASS FRAMES AND HAIRCUTS

Contoured Face Shapes

PEAR   Follow guidelines for round; however, fullness on top is necessary to broaden width of forehead.

   Hair should be kept close to face at cheek area. Bangs will often create the illusion of width.

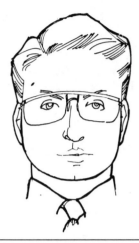

HEART   Follow guidelines for round, however fullness on bottom is necessary to balance narrow chin.

   Hair should be flat on side with some fullness in back to create the illusion of a fuller chin. An off-center part will cut width of forehead.

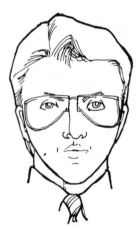

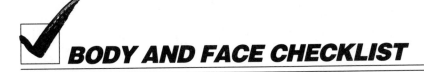

BODY AND FACE CHECKLIST

Getting to the top in style — a style that's yours alone — means cutting through the fads and fancies in clothing while developing a natural, custom-tailored look. Knowing and understanding your body shape and facial features is a big step toward that goal. You'll make the right choice every time and make your investment wardrobe purchases pay big dividends.

☐ Style doesn't change as fashion does. Define your personal style by selecting clothes that are a natural extension of your body line.

☐ Besides an extension of body line, flattering items need to complement your coloring and fit properly. Seek a balance between line, scale, and color.

☐ A man's body can be described in three basic shapes: sharp-straight, straight, and contoured. Facial features will generally conform to these shapes, too.

☐ Body lines remain consistent. Over the years, there may be some shifting and added weight. But, for the most part, the body line that defines you now will be the same in the future.

☐ The lines of clothing for men can be divided in two: the silhouette (the outline of a particular cut of suit), and detail lines (the little tailoring touches, such as pocket flaps and stitching). Of these, the silhouette is probably the most important consideration in making your selections.

☐ Don't fall into the trap of believing there are "ideal" body shapes. You may prefer to be thin or muscular, but ultimately any shape can be flattered, with your clothes accenting positive attributes and masking minor flaws.

☐ The shape of your face, like your body, is pretty much set for life. Knowing its geometry will help you achieve consistent style in your clothing selections. It will also show you which hairstyles and eyeglasses are right for you.

☐ Knowing what to look for in the basic men's suits — Brooks Brothers (Ivy League or "sack" style), modified American, and European cuts — is an invaluable way to formulate your own special look. The Brooks-type suit is softly contoured; the modified or updated American is a more angular, and the European cuts are most angular of all. Determine your particular body shape and go for the style and tailoring that's most natural.

☐ Double-check the face shapes in this chapter when you shop for shirts. In fact, take the book with you. The listing is guaranteed fool-proof. And it'll save you lots of money in the long run.

☐ Like any article of clothing, shirts follow the rule of "the Big A" — appropriateness. Button-downs are always fine for business; pin and bar collars are dressy; spread collars look best for European suits; round collars are dressy but unbusiness-like. Know when to apply the rules!

☐ Eyeglass frames and hairstyles must complement your face shapes. The suggestions listed will make costly mistakes a "has been."

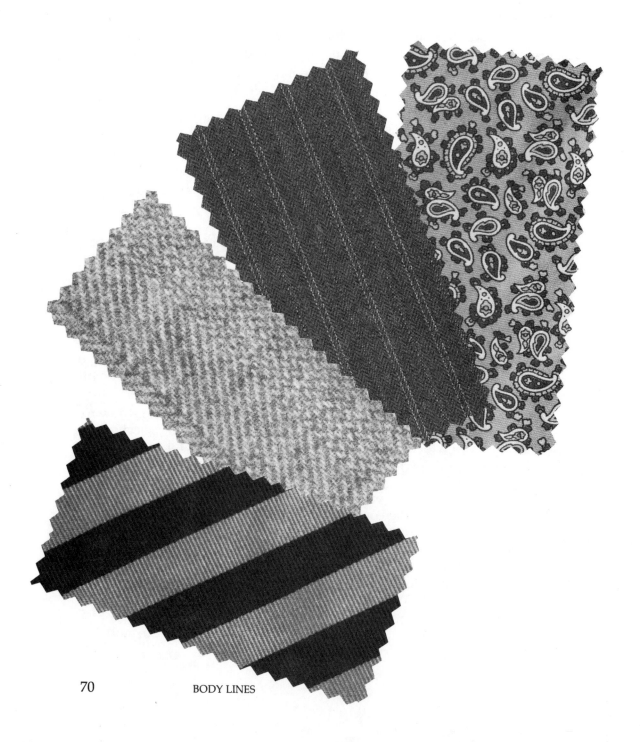

BODY LINES

CHAPTER FOUR

FABRICS AND DETAILS

A suit's silhouette is a primary definition of line. But there are other ways to make a line *straighter* or more contoured. The selection of fabric type is critical in defining a line.

Fabrics that are crisp, stiff, and tightly woven better define straight lines. Using softer fabrics relaxes a silhouette so that it complements the body shape with less exaggerated angles. Patterns and designs in the fabrics also make a difference. The pin-stripe, for example, projects a much straighter line than the softer chalk-stripe. Harris tweed is softer than herringbone. The crisp Glenn plaid is better for straight lines and a muted plaid in a soft wool flannel produces a more contoured shape.

The *details* of a suit are touches such as squared shoulder pads, angled pocket flaps, double-breasted jackets and well-defined "darts," a means of tucking in or opening up certain lines, such as the waist emphasis on a two-button suit jacket.

The world of fabrics and details could easily fill many libraries with technical volumes, few of which would be very useful outside of the fields of custom tailoring and the garment district. At Accolade, we've distilled the essentials and coordinated them with the various body shapes.

The following fabric types are best for the specific body lines:

Sharp-straight: Tightly woven; gabardine, worsted, sharkskin, linen, silk, also, crisp poplin, pin-stripes, crisp Glenn plaids, tightly woven herringbones; even check, or houndstooth check. Crisp geometric and abstract patterns with a sheen for neckties and sportswear patterns work best with these fabrics and lines.

Straight: Moderate to tightly woven; worsted, sharkskin, linen, flannel, cashmere, gabardine, herringbone, Glenn plaid, pin-stripe. Straight geometric patterns for neckties and sportswear or combinations of straight line designs are best.

Contoured: Softly woven; tweed, wood flannel, nubby texture, cashmere, matte finish, Glenn plaid in flannel, chalk-stripe. Patterns and designs that contain paisleys, swirls, or blended stripes work best for necktie and sportswear designs.

A Fabric Sampler

The following is a representative glossary of commonly used fabrics. It will help familiarize you with fabrics used in a wide variety of men's suits.

Broadcloth: A fine, closely woven, lustrous cotton or polyester/cotton fabric made in a plain weave with a fine rib. The cloth has a soft, firm finish.

Cashmere: A fine, soft, wool undergrowth produced by the Kashmir goat. It is often combined with silk, cotton, or wool. Uses: dresses, coats, and sweaters. It is a soft, elegant fabric with a slightly fuzzy surface. Good for contoured and some straight body types.

Chalk-stripe: Stripes resembling chalk lines. They project a softer appearance than pin-stripe. Good for contoured and some straight body lines.

Chino: Originally, chino was a slightly twilled fabric used for military uniforms. It is mercerized and Sanforized and today is used for sportswear.

Corduroy: A strong, durable fabric in which the rib has been sheared or woven to produce a smooth, velvet-like nap with wide or narrow wales, cords, or ribs. May be of cotton, polyester, rayon or blends.

Denim: A well-known basic cotton or blended fabric. Right or left-handed twill constructions, usually in the latter weave. Generally the warp is dyed blue with a white filling. The fabric is very durable and is popular for all types of garments from work clothes to sportswear and evening wear. Variation in structural design and coloring has increased the demand for denim in the fashion fabric field since the 1970's. Pre-washed versions are best for contoured body types.

End-on-End: An arrangement of warp yarns with one end of color and one end of white alternately. The filling is generally white or a solid color. This type of construction is used widely in men's suit and underwear fabrics and women's and children's washable garments. Creates a grainy, almost checkered look. Contoured-straight.

HOW FABRIC CAN EFFECT
THE CHARACTER OF A GARMENT

*Best Cut for
Sharp-Straight
Body Shape*

*Best Cut for
Straight
Body Shape*

*Best Cut for
Contoured
Body Shape*

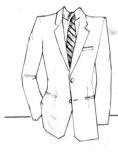

In a softer fabric
will work for the
Straight body shape. →

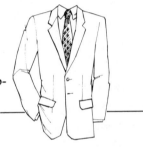

← In a crisper fabric
will work for the Sharp-
Straight body shape.

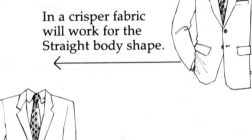

← In a crisper fabric
will work for the
Straight body shape.

In a softer fabric
will work for the
Contoured body shape. →

Yᴏᴜ have options. Your first step is to identify your body shape and learn to identify which of the three basic cuts of suit is going to be your bet. By applying the information in *Successful Style* on the way fabrics affect the look of a garment, you'll discover other cuts you may be able to wear.

Flannel: A loosely woven fabric with a soft nap. It is primarily made of wool or cotton. Contoured-straight.

Foulard: (*foo-lard*) A lightweight, soft fabric of twill or plain weave popular for neckties and scarves. A foulard print refers to small all-over patterns like those used traditionally on men's neckties.

Gabardine: Tightly woven, twill fabric. Best for sharp-straight and straight.

Glenn check: Glenn patterns usually consist of checks in varying colors with overlines or overchecks of other colors. Glenn check and glenn plaids are the same.

Harris Tweed: This name refers to woolens handwoven on the islands of the Outer Hebrides off the northern coast of Scotland. Loosely woven, nubby. Best for contoured.

Herringbone: A twill weave in which the weave reverses so the twill pattern forms a ''V'' pattern. It is also called broken twill houndstooth. (See Check).

A zigzag woven pattern suggesting the skeleton of a fish. Rows of chevron stripes are woven in two contrasting or close colors to form this pattern. For all body lines depending on the lightness of the weave.

Hopsack: Coarse and loosely woven fabric with basket-weave effect. Used for suits, jackets, and slacks. Best for contoured.

Houndstooth check: A pointed, broken check, regular in pattern.

Oxford cloth: Oxford cloth is most often used to describe a basket or plain weave fabric made of cotton or cotton blend. It often has a colored warp and a white filling. This fabric is given a smooth finish and is a popular fabric for men's shirts. It is the one remaining important commercial shirting variety of four originally made by a Scotch mill in the late 19th century, which have the names of four universities, Oxford, Cambridge, Harvard, and Yale.

Paisley: Paisley is usually used to describe a design made in Paisley, Scotland. The shawls were originally woven to imitate the shawls of Kahsmir which had a cone design. The woven shawls proved too expensive to produce and the design was adopted for printing. The Paisley design itself changed to the scroll-like form it now has.

Pin stripe: A fine, slender stripe on a fabric, approximately the width of a straight pin. Term also refers to a fabric with such a stripe.

Poplin: A durable, plain weave class of fabric having fine cross ribs. Made of silk, cotton, manmade fibers, wool, etc., or a combination of these fibers. Similar to broadcloth, but with a heavier rib. The fabric known as cotton broadcloth shirting in the U.S. was developed in Great Britain and known there as poplin.

Silk: Continuous protein filament produced by the larvae of the silkworm (Bomoyx mori) when constructing their cocoons. The filament is reeled off and oiled to remove a stiff natural glue, and woven into fabrics noted for their soft luster, luxurious hand, and strength.

Tattersall check: Tattersall checks are an overcheck pattern in two colors, usually on a white or other colored ground. An example would be a pattern of brown lines going in one direction crossed by green lines in the opposite direction, forming the checks on a yellow background.

Tweed: A rough-surfaced wool fabric of two or more colors. Tightly woven will work for straight and sharp-straight.

Twill: A basic weave characterized by a diagonal rib, or twill line, generally running upward from left to right. Twill weaves are used to produce a strong, durable, firm fabric. They can be varied in many ways, e.g., broken, herringbone, etc.

Worsted: A very smooth-surfaced wool fabric woven of worsted (twisted) yarn spun from long-staple, evenly combed wool. Can be used by all body types.

As mentioned, this is a quick sampling. Keep in mind that continuity must be maintained between suit fabric and the selection of shirts and ties. The fabrics and patterns should work together, so that the lines of each works with the suit. More on shirts and ties later. More geometric designs project straighter lines. The tighter woven fabrics create straighter lines. Softer weaves soften the silhouette line.

Describing Your Facial Features

Facial characteristics are defined differently. Cheeks, nose shapes and mouth and chin sizes are described as being *broad*, *average*, or *fine*.

These terms are critical to making successful clothing choices.

The words carry no subjective or judgmental overtones. They're used to determine which fabrics and details go best with your shape and style and give you a balanced appearance. This is how it works:

Large bones, broad facial features: These men should select heavier-weight fabrics, accessories, and eyeglass frames. The lighter weights make it appear as if you overpower your clothing.

Small bones, average to fine facial features: Stay away from heavy fabrics, frames, and accessories. Your clothes will overpower you.

Look at the drawing of the two blazers in the chart entitled *How fabric weight effects the character of a garment*. You'll notice that one of them is drawn with a fine-tipped pen, indicating a light-weight fabric. The other is drawn with a broad-tipped pen, indicating a heavier look that would be more balanced on someone with larger bone structure.

HOW FABRIC WEIGHT EFFECTS THE CHARACTER OF A GARMENT

Light Weight Fabric   *Heavy Weight Fabric*

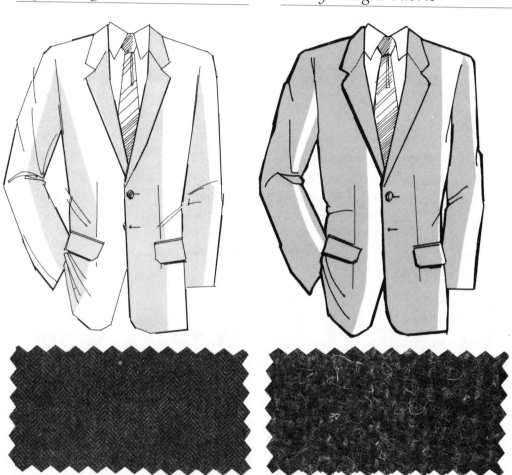

Men with large bones and broad facial features should choose heavier-weight fabrics, accessories and eyeglass frames. Lighter weight elements will make it appear as if you overpower your clothing.

Men with small bones and average to fine facial features should choose more finely woven fabrics and smaller scaled accessories. These will prevent clothing from overpowering you.

Fabrics come in all weights. It's only necessary to look and feel the materials to recognize the differences. To be aware of such details helps clue you in as to why you may be more comfortable with certain outfits now in your closet.

Fabric and Your Bone Structure

Your bone structure and muscle define your body and facial characteristics — your basic physical structure. The structure may be large, small, or in between. How do you know for sure where you fit in?

Look at your wrists. When you circle your wrist with your thumb and index fingers, how much space is left over between them? If you're small-boned, you'll have about a half-inch left over. If you happen to be medium-size, you'll have about an inch-wide gap between your thumb and index finger. If there's more than an inch left over, consider yourself large-boned.

If you're right-handed, measure your left (less-developed wrist). Left-handers should try it on their right wrist. Similar measurements may also be taken on your ankles.

The Best Fabrics for Businesswear

While there isn't an absolute rule about which fabrics fit in best on the job, certain unspoken traditions have evolved. These have mostly to do with the look and feel projected by certain fabrics and blends. Perhaps the most obvious aspect is that some fabrics have a "richer" look than others; in a quiet way they have an "executive" aura.

The most recommended for a business setting are 100 percent wool, wool blends, cotton blends, silk, linen, and linen blends.

It's generally agreed that the best blends are 55 percent or more of natural fibers and 45 percent or less of manmade fiber. In the past, *only* natural fibers were recommended for serious suits and other articles of clothing. These days, however, this point of view has changed. Given the progress made in the use of synthetics and the excellent blends that have been made available to the general market, the *natural fibers only* admonition has softened.

It's become a matter of personal choice. Natural materials are cooler in warm weather, and some men prefer the feel. Other men like the blends because they're easy to care for. Either way, comfort and fit are foremost. Be aware, however, that your style isn't going to be advanced by what looks to all the world like a "plastic suit" — a totally synthetic job. Technology may eventually come up with a synthetic offering that equals — or even exceeds in quality — the naturals. In the meantime, go for all-natural fibers, or quality blends.

Best Fabrics for Sharp-Straight Bodies

☐ **Body lines to look for:** sharp-straight silhouette, angular face shape, exaggerated shoulders.

☐ **Fabrics:** tightly woven, little or no texture, crisp.

HOW TEXTURE CAN EFFECT THE CHARACTER OF A GARMENT

Tightly Woven Fabric   *Textured, Loosely Woven Fabric*

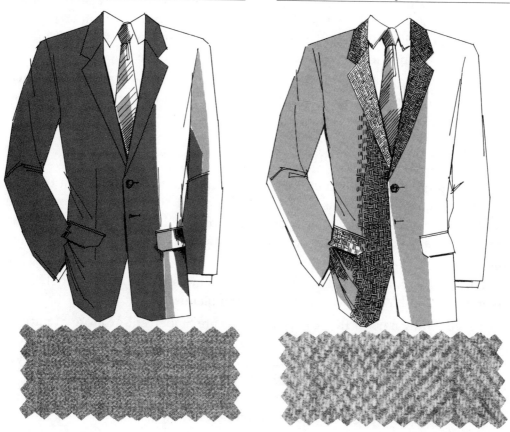

By using a softer, more loosely woven fabric, the silhouette line of the garment is softened.

Fabric types:
- Suits: gabardine, linen, twill, silk, worsted, sharkskin.
- Shirts: broadcloth, pinpoint, silk.
- Ties: silk.
- Patterns: geometric, abstract, sharp plaids, checks, herringbone, houndstooth, pin-stripes.

A garment's silhouette becomes sharper when tightly woven, crisp fabrics are used.

☐ **Ties:** solid, stripe, geometric, abstract, pin dot, sharp paisley.

Best Fabrics for Straight Bodies

☐ **Body lines to look for:** straight silhouette, rectangular face shape, square shoulders.

☐ **Fabrics:** moderate to tightly woven, some texture.

Fabric types:
- Suits: gabardine, worsted, flannel, cashmere, silk, linen.
- Shirts: broadcloth, pin-point, oxford cloth.
- Ties: silk, wool.
- Patterns: pin-stripe, herringbone, Glenn plaid, checks.

As a garment's silhouette becomes straighter, be sure you compensate with a slightly softer fabric such as flannel, worsted, cashmere, which will soften the line.

☐ **Ties:** solid, stripes, polka dot, club, foulard.

Best Fabrics for Contoured Bodies

☐ **Body lines to look for:** rectangular silhouette, contoured face shape, sloping shoulders.

☐ **Fabrics:** soft textures, loosely woven, nubby finish, dull or matte finish.

Fabric types:
- Suit: worsted, flannel, cashmere, basket weave, linen.
- Shirt: broadcloth, oxford cloth, end-on-end.
- Tie: silk, wool, knit.
- Patterns: Glenn plaid (blended), herringbone, chalk stripe, tweed.

As a garment's silhouette becomes straighter, be sure you compensate with a softer fabric such as flannel, worsted, or cashmere which will soften the line.

☐ **Ties:** solid, blended stripe, club, foulards, paisley.

Combining Suits, Shirts and Ties

Now that you know what fabrics and patterns are best for your body line, it is important to understand how to combine your suit, shirt, and ties. There is much flexibility when considering personalities and fashion trends. Recently, more color and pattern mixing is being used in the men's industry. As with the other guidelines offered so far, the rules for combination are based on conservative, safe, and complementary uses of design and pattern mixing in a corporate environment where classic is correct.

General guidelines:
- Shirts should be lighter than the suit
- Ties darker than the shirt
- Only two color families should be used, i.e., navy suit, blue shirt, and navy tie with red or other complementary color. (White shirts do not count as a color). Avoid navy suit, yellow shirt, and gray and burgundy tie.

Combining patterns:
- Three solids
- One solid and two patterns
- Two solids and one pattern
- Combining three patterns gives a less conservative, more fashion forward look. It can be done successfully but takes skill and experience. Avoid it unless you are confident of your ability and/or use a personal shopper.

See charts in this chapter for different body lines.

 # SUIT, SHIRT AND TIE COMBINATIONS FOR THE SHARP-STRAIGHT BODY LINE

☐ **Solid Suit**
- **With a solid shirt-tie patterns:** Solid, Stripe, Foulard (geometric), Polka dot (pin), Crisp paisley.
- **With a pin-stripe shirt-tie patterns:** Solid, Stripe, Foulard (geometric), Polka dot (pin), crisp paisley.

☐ **Pin Stripe Suit**
- **With a solid shirt-tie patterns:** Solid, Stripe, Foulard (geometric), Polka dot (pin), Crisp paisley.

THE RIGHT PATTERNS FOR YOUR TIES

Sharp-Straight

SOLID

STRIPE

ABSTRACT

PIN DOT

GEOMETRIC

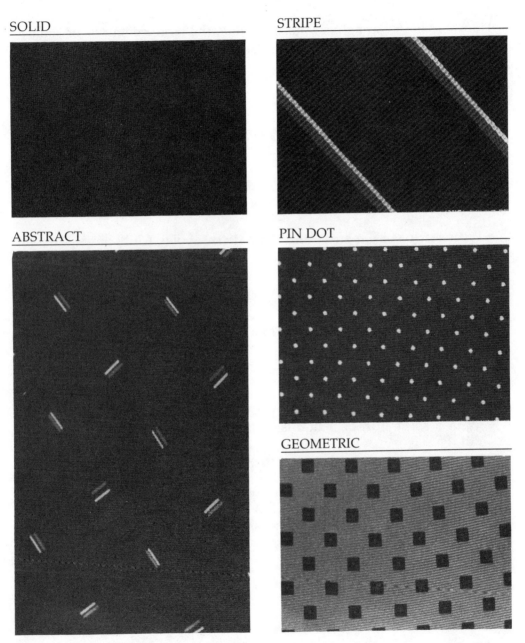

The man with a Sharp-Straight face should look for crisp patterns, made up of straight lines in tightly woven fabrics. Shiny and smooth fabrics create sharper lines.

- **With a different width pin-stripe shirt-tie pattern:** Solid.
- ☐ **Crisp Glenn Plaid Suit**
  - **With a solid shirt-tie patterns:** Solid, Stripe, Foulard (geometric), Polka dot (pin), Crisp paisley.

The sharper and straighter your body line, the more geometric or "sharp" your tie patterns should be. When selecting a tie avoid very loosely woven soft fabrics.

✓ SUIT, SHIRT AND TIE COMBINATIONS FOR THE STRAIGHT BODY LINE

☐ **Solid Suit**
  - **With a solid shirt-tie patterns:** Solid, Club, Stripe, Foulard, Pin polka dot, Paisley.
  - **With a stripe or pin-stripe shirt-tie patterns:** Solid, Club, Stripe, Foulard, Pin polka dot.

☐ **Pin-stripe Suit**
  - **With a solid shirt-tie patterns:** Solid, Club, Stripe, Foulard, Pin polka dot, Paisley.
  - **With a stripe or pin-stripe shirt of a different width-tie pattern:** Solid.

☐ **Glenn Plaid Suit**
  - **With a solid shirt-tie patterns:** Solid, Club, Stripe, Foulard, Pin polka dot.

☐ **Herringbone Suit**
  - **With a solid shirt-tie patterns:** Solid, Club, Stripe, Foulard, Pin polka dot, Paisley.
  - **With a stripe or pin-stripe shirt-tie pattern:** Solid.

If your body type is straight, rectangular, or square, avoid extremes of sharpness or curviness in patterns. When selecting a tie, avoid extremes available . . . choose neither very loosely woven - soft, nor tightly woven - very crisp fabrics.

THE RIGHT PATTERNS FOR YOUR TIES

Straight

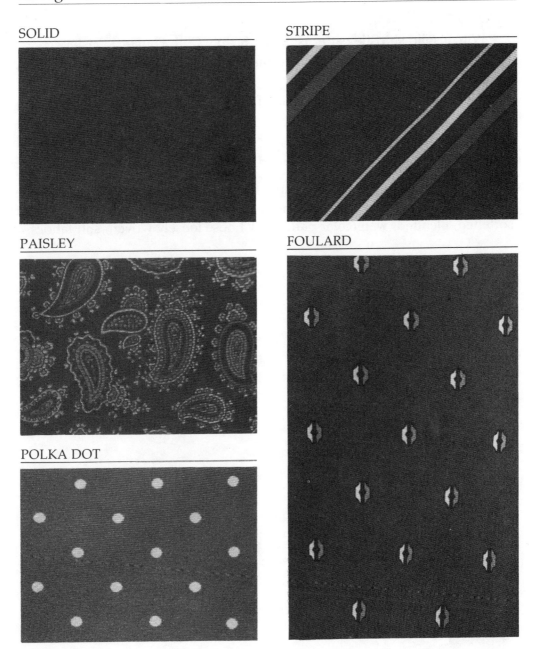

SOLID

STRIPE

PAISLEY

FOULARD

POLKA DOT

The man with a Straight face should avoid extremes of very crisp or very loosely woven fabrics, and extremes of very crisp or blended patterns.

SUIT, SHIRT AND TIE COMBINATIONS FOR THE CONTOUR BODY LINE

☐ **Solid Suit**
- With a solid shirt-tie patterns: Solid, Stripe, Club Foulard, Paisley.
- With a oxford-stripe shirt-tie patterns: Solid, Stripe, Club, Foulard, Paisley.

☐ **Chalk-Stripe Suit**
- With a solid shirt-tie patterns: Solid, Stripe, Club, Foulard, Paisley.
- With a stripe of a different width-tie pattern: Solid.

☐ **Glenn Plaid Suit**
- With a solid shirt-tie patterns: Solid, Stripe, Club, Foulard, Paisley.

The more contoured your body line, the less geometric or "sharp" your tie patterns should be. When selecting a tie, avoid crisp patterns in favor of softened, blended, watercolor patterns. Choose loosely woven, soft fabrics.

THE RIGHT PATTERNS FOR YOUR TIES

Contoured

SOLID

BLENDED STRIPE

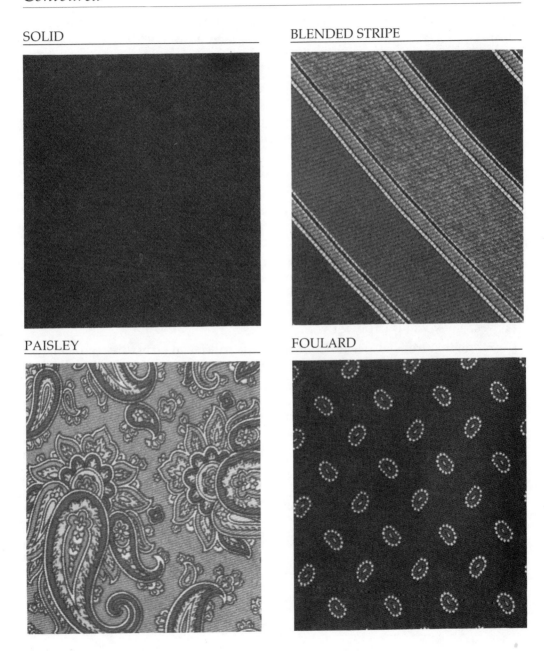

PAISLEY

FOULARD

The man with a Contoured face shouls look for blended, watercolor patterns with curved lines in soft fabrics. Matte finish or textured fabrics create softer lines.

✔ FABRICS AND PATTERNS: A CHECKLIST

Fabrics and details are critical to complementing body and even facial shape, emphasizing straight and contoured lines, as required. This list provides the summary data you need to make smart choices.

☐ For straight lines, think fabrics that are crisp, stiff and tightly woven. Contoured lines are flattered by soft loosely woven materials.

☐ As fabric selections are softened, shoulder treatment, pocket styles, darts, and other "details" tend to be more relaxed.

☐ Patterns and designs also make a difference in line. The pin stripe, for example, projects a straight line, while chalk- stripe is best for contoured features.

☐ Continuity in fabric and design needs to be maintained. Lines must work together — from suit, to shirt, to necktie. You needn't "match" everything; just make sure that combination flows naturally.

☐ Check your bone structure and determine if it's large, medium, or small. See if your facial features are broad, average or fine. Balance fabrics and details to achieve harmony and style.

☐ Small-boned, fine-featured men should stay away from heavy weight fabrics. They will overpower your features.

☐ Fabric texture is also a function of body and facial structure. Smaller men look best in light textures; the bulkier items work best for medium to larger bodies.

☐ Take time out to study fabrics and textures. Both are important but too little understood. They can make a big difference in the way you look and feel in your clothing.

☐ For businesswear, the most accepted materials are 100 percent wool, wool and cotton blends, silk, linen and linen blends. The best blends are 55 percent or more natural fibers, 45 percent or less manmade fibers.

☐ Be careful in your use of synthetics. Avoid the blatantly "plastic suit." It downgrades your style.

☐ Proper combining of patterns and fabrics create the finishing touches for a pulled together look.

FABRICS FOR YOUR SUITS

Sharp-Straight

The best fabrics for the
Sharp-Straight body
lines are crisp, tightly
woven and have little or
no texture.

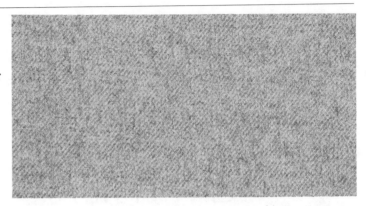

Straight

The best fabrics for the
Straight body line are
moderately to tightly
woven and have some
texture.

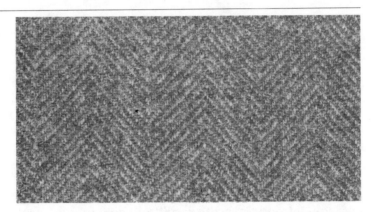

Contoured

The best fabrics for the
Contoured body line are
loosely woven, softly
textured, nubby, dull or
matte finish.

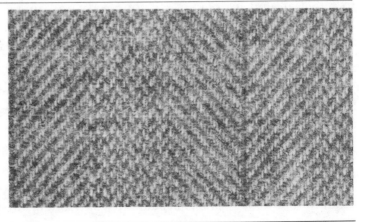

CHAPTER FIVE

••

FIT AND QUALITY

Only Great Will Do

*I*t's called "scale" — fitting clothes perfectly to your body shape. It's a cut that, in all details, looks like it was made for you.

Scale is the essential difference between looking ordinary and elegant. Not foppish elegance, but quiet good taste. It's amazing that this #10-size secret of dressing well isn't universally known. Fit — fit and good materials. If you achieve it, what you get is consistency, quality, simplicity, and comfort. Elegance.

Warning: Fit has a downside.

If you insist on being tightly fitted (the macho guy!) or if you want the tailor to give you a trendy cut, the result will be very *unelegant*.

Most tailored suits fit the body in an easy, natural way. There's plenty of room to move around in, perfect for your body and shape, without being overly loose. This gives you an expensive look. If you're thin, this cut will make you look a little heavier. And if you're heavy, it'll make you look 10 pounds lighter.

Of course, none of this is easy. Buying the right suit and getting the proper fit is expensive and time consuming. Prices run from $250 up to $800 or $1000. Given the stakes, it's definitely worthy of your best efforts.

Don't assume that the sizing of your last suit will automatically translate to your new purchases. Bodies change and proper fitting requires that you take all the time you need to do it right.

One of our Always In Style clients gave us a good illustration of how assumptions about your vital statistics can work against you.

After graduation from college some years ago, our client found himself only a few days away from an important job interview. On borrowed cash, he headed for the best men's store in town, where he purchased one of the most expensive suits on the rack. It was a beauty: a gray wool blend with fine construction and detailing. The clerk beamed, "Good choice, sir." As it happened, the tailor was at lunch and the clerk urged the buyer to return for a fitting.

"That won't be necessary," our client replied. He'd purchased many suits and he knew his measurements. He wrote them on a slip of paper, to be given later to the tailor.

"You may be making a mistake," the clerk responded.

"Trust me," our client said.

A few days later when the suit was ready our client stood in front of a full-length mirror at home and tried it on. That's when it hit him. The trousers were too short, the waist too snug, and the jacket hung like a Roman toga.

"Somebody goofed!" he told himself.

Indeed, someone had goofed, and the image of that person was staring back at him from the mirror.

He had made a common error. He hadn't taken into account the natural shifting of one's body shape over time. The result was that this beautiful, expensive suit looked as if he had outgrown it. Fortunately, the tailor worked overtime to correct the problems, adding to the expense. He wore it to the interview and he did get the job — but it was a close call.

Fit and Quality Checkpoints

Price isn't everything, especially when it comes to the right fit. No matter how much you pay for an item of clothing, if the fit isn't there, then everything else suffers. Poor fit makes a $1000 suit look cheap and the highest quality will seem only shoddy.

Most fine stores employ one or more tailors, but it's up to you to understand the possibilities you see reflected in the fitting room mirror. It's a bit like taking your car in for repairs: If you don't understand the engine and what may be wrong with it, you're at the mercy of indifferent forces. This isn't to imply that tailors are indifferent; they aren't, and, for the most part, they take a lot of pride in their work. Still it's best if you can communicate and, to some extent, guide the tailoring process.

What follows are the basics of good fit:

Suit and Sport Jackets

- No wrinkles across the back or under the collar.
- Jacket should cover your buttocks. The most useful formula is to measure the length from the collar seam all the way to the floor and divide in half. This isn't fool-proof, so check to make sure the tailor knows what you're looking for by way of length.
- The jacket sleeve should be at the wristbone with your arms at your side. When your curl your arms, the sleeve shouldn't rise more than a quarter-inch above this point.
- Handsewn interfacing is preferable. Fused and ironed-on tailoring should be avoided if possible.
- Hand finishing gives a garment a rich look. Insist on this fine point when selecting a jacket.
- Make sure all top stitching is even. No loose ends!
- Your sleeves should have button holes, either real ones or imitations.
- Don't overlook buttons. They should be made of bone, not plastic.
- On a sport jacket, the use of leather or metal is perfectly acceptable. But not on a traditional suit.
- Fabric must be a natural fiber or a quality blend.

Trousers

It's extra important that your trousers be well-cut and comfortable. You may take off your jacket as soon as you get to the office, but the trousers are with you for the rest of the day. The best fit is one that feels as if the material isn't there at all. What follows are some insider tailoring tips to help achieve maximum ease and comfort.

- Trouser legs should break in front over the tops of your shoes. No draggers and no high waters!
- The legs should be tapered toward the back, ending where shoe and heel connect.
- If the pockets flair out when you try on the trousers, they're probably too tight. Pockets should be flat and even in a good fit.
- Same goes for pleats. If they flair, the pants are too snug. Pleats must be comfortably folded and easy looking.
- Trousers should fall straight from the buttocks.
- Suit trousers should have belt loops for belt. If you're going to wear them with suspenders, have the tailor sew good, solid buttons inside the waistband to

accommodate them and eliminate belt loops. The fit of the waist should be looser for suspenders.

● Long-legged men may wear trouser cuffs; shorter men will look better without cuffs.

THE TEN BIGGEST MISTAKES IN GETTING A SUIT THAT FITS

When a suit has the "right" cut, it looks like it was made for you. It is perfect for your body shape. However, it must also fit properly.

The proper fit can be identified as "elegantly loose." It will make you look thinner if you are too heavy, heavier if you are too thin. Most importantly, the wrong fit can make an otherwise perfect suit look inexpensive regardless of its cost.

There are basic rules to follow in selecting a suit that fits you perfectly—all are listed in Chapter Five. But here are the ten mistakes men most commonly make.

1. Jacket sleeve too short

2. Jacket length too short

3. Jacket wrinkles across back, below collar

4. Buckled or wrinkled lapel when jacket is closed

5. Wrinkles at arm hole seam

6. Trouser too short

7. Pleats and pockets pull open

8. Waist too tight

9. Too high or too low rise in trouser

10. Trouser hem not tapered toward back

● In trying on and wearing trousers, don't let the waistband fall below your stomach. Wear them at the waistline or a little below it, at the top of your hips. Allow two fingers to fit in the waistband.

Shirts

● Sleeves should extend 1/4-1/2'' from jacket sleeve.

● No short-sleeve shirts under suits or sport jackets.

● Allow one finger to fit in collar.

● Buttons must remain closed with one-inch allowance on side and under arm.

● Should be long enough to stay tucked in neatly.

Communicating With Your Tailor

For most of us, it's hard to appreciate the deadline pressure imposed on most tailors, especially those working for large menswear outlets. During any given day they'll be called upon to fit a dozen or more gentlemen, almost all of whom will insist on a rush job.

Under the circumstances, it's a good idea to tell the tailor how to proceed; let him know which details are important in fitting your body. Some tailors — like certain auto mechanics — may resent your self-interest. No matter. After all, you're paying the tab. For the most part, however, good fitters will appreciate a little guidance. It's a bit like signing a contract: Everybody knows what's expected of them. It makes the job that much easier.

Below are some tips that will help assure a first-rate fitting.

● The way a pant leg breaks on your shoe top depends on the heel. Always wear your business shoes during a fitting. This will assure a proper break, since the height of the heel will be factored in exactly.

● When being fitted, assume a normal posture. Many men make the mistake of standing at attention in front of the mirror. It's an unnatural pose and it will make a difference in fit. Stand normally, at ease. If the tailor insists on your coming to attention, let him know you're not buying a military uniform. The suit needs to conform to your natural stance.

● Will the suit shrink or lose its shape at the laundry? Read any labels and confirm the information with the fitter.

● To be certain the sleeves will be cut to the proper length, make it a point to wear a long-sleeved dress shirt when trying on the jacket. If you wear French cuffs, bring them along. Remember: one-quarter to one-half inch of cuff should show.

● Most tailors automatically hem trousers without a cuff. If you want a cuff, say so.

● It's okay to ask a tailor questions about what goes with the suit you're buying. Tie, shoes, belts, shirts — it's all part of the game. In the end, it's up to you. Practice, practice, practice. Develop your sense of color, line, and style, because if you really want it done right you'll simply have to resolve to do it yourself!

Is There An 'Ideal' Body Shape?

Until the dawn of the "Me Generation" of the 1970's, women maintained an uncomfortable corner on the notion of strutting an "ideal" body. Since that era, men have joined women in the pervasive hype that seems to insist that all of us look like 18-year-olds.

Chances are that women are forever trapped by physical ideals. It's unfair, it's unreal, but it's also here to stay. Men, on the other hand, aren't quite so locked in. Wisely they resist the barrage of stereotypes that fly at them from all directions, including the world of fashion. Women should resist, too, but this remains for a more enlightened future generation.

If an historical "ideal" exists for men, it focuses on a physique with shoulders that are 10 inches larger than the hips. That's fine if your DNA has cooperated, but, for the most part, men are indifferent — and rightly so — to such stereotyping. More than ever before they are aware of fitness and health, and certainly their sense of good looks is on the upswing. But as for "ideal" bodies, forget it!

The real concern is making the most of what you've got. To this noble end, we offer the following tips:

Contoured bodies: These men look terrific in light-colored sport coats made of soft and loosely woven fabrics. In casual wear, darker trousers will create the look of more narrow hips. Crisp or stiff fabrics should be avoided.

Pattern or tweed sport jackets also work. Some padding is needed in the shoulders, but not to the point of producing large, square shoulders.

On the casual side, the contoured man will look great in bulky, "fisherman" of Fair Isle sweaters worn with solid slacks.

Horizontal stripes for sport shirts and sweaters work well, especially muted, blended, or uneven stripes that keep the line softened. Boat-neck sweaters are also excellent.

The contoured man should avoid V-necks and raglan sleeves.

Muscular, rectangular bodies, with little fat: This is a straight body line leaning slightly in the direction of being contoured.

These bodies require absolutely no camouflage. This is the shape around which most designers build their clothing lines. Color and pattern varieties are infinite. Some shoulder emphasis is desirable, but not critical.

Broad shoulders, narrow hips (sharp-straight body): This group can easily wear double-breasted jackets. Little or no shoulder padding is required.

These men should go for flatter, tightly woven fabrics for suits and jackets. As for sweaters, V-neck and turtle-neck types are excellent choices.

Stripes also work well. However, sharp straight men should avoid paisley or heather patterned sweaters and tight-fitting shirts.

Tall and thin, next to no body fat: This is the straight body line with typically small bone structure.

A looser fit adds some weight to this body shape. Be aware, however, that a contrasting jacket and slacks will make you look shorter than you really are.

On trousers, cuffs are preferred.

Avoid heavy fabrics. If you want to look stronger, opt for light to medium weights.

Slight padding in the shoulders of suits and sport jackets fill out the figure, and vests add bulk to your overall appearance. Overplaids and plaids, especially, give a feeling of extra breadth. Crisp Glenn plaids are best. Horizontal stripes, boat-neck, and crew neck seaters are good sportswear choices.

Short men: These men need to use the same clothing lines as those outlined for their body lines. Proper scale and texture is critical.

Short men should stay away from strong contrasts.

Vertical patterns (pin and chalk stripes) work best.

Choose a slightly narrower tie than the standard three-and-a-quarter inch/three-and-a-half-inch models.

Trousers should continue in an unbroken line to the floor, uncuffed, with a slight break at the top of the shoe.

Don't sacrifice the total look of quality, fit, and line to make yourself look a half-inch taller. Be especially careful to select fabrics and a silhouette consistent with your body line.

Round, prominent abdomen, fleshy, short-limbed: You'll look better in chalk stripes or solids, and single-breasted suits are better looking than double-breasted models.

Shoulders should be slightly padded. Worsted wool or wool flannel is better looking than tightly woven fabrics.

Minimal contrast should be maintained between jackets and slacks, and soft fabrics work better than bulky offerings.

It's best to avoid cuffed trousers, and the sleeve length of jackets should be slightly longer than the break of the wrist.

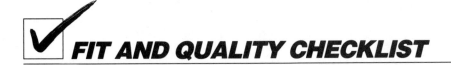

FIT AND QUALITY CHECKLIST

When considering the purchase of expensive outfits, it's best to have all the information and tips you can muster going in. You may want to take this checklist with you on your next foray to the menswear store.

☐ "Scale" — the fitting of clothes to your particular body shape — is the difference between looking super and looking ordinary — or less! Your best bet is a loose (not baggy) fit. Stay away from tight fits. Besides looking bizarre, the tightly fitted suit will be useless the moment your proportions change.

☐ Go with your current vital statistics. Chances are that last year's measurements have changed. Be aware of this and insist on being measured for the way you are *now*.

☐ Carefully examine the proportions of the three basic suits: natural shoulder, modified American, and the European cut. Don't try to force yourself into any model that tends to exaggerate your lines. (See page 11 of this chapter).

☐ Beware the "athletic cut." Unless you're a hard-core jock and/or body builder, this trendy style probably won't enhance your classic look.

☐ The retailers and manufacturers are forever pushing new styles. It's a critical element of their economies. The question is: Why should you be the one to take a risk? Don't worry about what's supposed to be "in." Trends change overnight, and investment clothes buying resists such volatility.

☐ If you're stocky or portly, stick with wool blends, solid colors, and pinstripes. If you're muscular, take the same advice. Stick to simplicity. Slender men should wear heavier fabrics and will look fine in a variety of patterns.

☐ When trying on a suit or a jacket or a pair of trousers, bring your normal shirt and shoes with you. This will help in bringing in the very best fit. Consider how the new article will be worn and where.

☐ At your next fitting bring the list of checkpoints on page 11 along with you. You want to make sure all the small details — collar, cuffs, break of the pant leg — are perfect for you.

☐ Communicate with your tailor. Tell him exactly what you want and need. Ask for input, but know in advance the kind of quality and fit you're looking for.

☐ If the fit isn't right, let the store know it on the spot. Don't hang that expensive suit in your closet until you're totally happy with the result.

CHAPTER SIX

PERSONAL STYLE

What's Perfect For You?

*I*t's time to put everything in order using the information and insight you've gained from the previous chapters.

In this chapter, we've matched body types (contoured, straight, and sharp-straight) with two basic looks, or occasions: your business look (what's best for you at the office) and a casual look for off-hours and leisure times.

Obviously none of these charts are cast in store. There may be variations, depending on the individual and your perception of total personal style. That's one of the nice things about these charts; they allow for your input. No one develops great personal style or panache dressing by the numbers!

Yet having the numbers in front of you can be a significant advantage. The charts are practical, and they will provide a baseline, a solid jumping off point from which you can add dashes of individuality.

How do you do it?

One way is to understand which items of clothing reflect your personality most directly. In the United States a man's necktie is a minor mirror of his soul. Up to a point it's a "free space" in which to express your personality. Think about it. When others compliment your clothing, it's most often your tie that receives first mention, followed by your suit. Shirts typically rank third, which puts them in the "honorable mention" category.

The point is that the five ties that go with solid suits on contoured bodies *require your personalized touch*. Yes, a club tie looks terrific with a blue suit, but it's up to you to get just the right color and design that says something about your personality.

While dressing by the numbers is okay, it's a little too safe not to be sorry at some point down the road. So by all means be a little daring, a little personal. Color your wardrobe in the same ways you color the world around you — by a direct projection of personal taste and style.

A Gallery of "IT" Men

Remember Clara Bow? She was the fabulous "IT" girl of the silent screen of the 1920's. Though it's hard to compare her to anyone of more recent vintage, it wouldn't be stretching too far to suggest that she was the Marilyn Monroe of her day.

"IT" was the most intriguing aspect of her personality because the word was so incredibly suggestive. Clara Bow's "IT" was variously translated to mean "sexy," "chic," "perky," "romantic," "amusing." Any adjective seemed to fit.

"IT" was certainly not confined to Clara Bow or females generally. The Great Lover, Rudolph Valentino, also possessed "IT." So did Douglas Fairbanks. And, more recently, a few of our more celebrated "IT" men include Miami Vice here Don Johnson, actor George C. Scott, musician David Sandborne, comic David Letterman, leader Lee Iacocca, on-again/off-again Middleweight Champion "Sugar Ray" Leonard, and Vulcan cult hero, Leonard Nimoy.

There are others from all walks of life — "IT" men that capture the imagination all the way to the bank and beyond. They've made it, or are in the process of making it, to the top. To them, and to those around them, "IT" means style, individuality, an intangible something that draws others to them. They get the breaks, and they know how to make the most of them.

You, too, have "IT." And it begins with the charts on the following pages. Please use them as a guide and, as indicated earlier, as a platform to develop your uniqueness.

✔ SHARP-STRAIGHT BODY AND CLOTHING LINES

☐ **Face Shape:**
- Square
- Diamond
- Rectangular

☐ **Body Shape:**
- Triangular
- Exaggerated Shoulders

☐ **Overall Impression:**
- Angularity
- Sharp-straight lines

☐ **Bone Structure and Body Proportion:**
- Small-Average 5'9''
- Average 5'10'' to 6'1''
- Average-Large 6'2'' or over

YOUR BUSINESS LOOK

- Suits

  Style: European cut (padded shoulders, waist emphasis), Updated American, Single-breasted, Double-breasted, Peaked lapel (sharp notch).

  Fabric: Tightly woven, Gabardine, Worsted, Sharksin, Pinstripe: 1/8'' - 1/4'' - 1/2'', Linen, Silk, Slight sheen, Crisp Glenn plaid, Crisp poplin, Solid color.

- Dress Shirts

  Style: Tapered fit, Pin collar, Standard collar, Spread collar, Contrasting collar and cuffs.

  Fabric: Broadcloth, Silk, Pin point, Stripe (pin), Solid.

- Ties

  Design: Solid, Stripe, Geometric or abstract, Polka dot (pin), Crisp paisley.

  Fabric: Silk, Raw silk, Shiny.

- Shoes

  Tie, Plain slip-on, Thin sole.

- Top Coat

  Style: Trench (epaulets), Double-breasted, Peaked lapel, Notched lapel, Set-in sleeve, Set-in or slash pocket.

  Fabric: Twill, Gabardine, Cashmere (with emphasized straight lines), Linen, Poplin, Crisp denim.

YOUR CASUAL LOOK

☐ **Sport Coat**

  Style: European cut (shoulder, and waist emphasis), Double-breasted, Single-breasted, Notched lapel, Peaked lapel, No top-stiching.

  Fabric: Tightly woven, Gabardine, Worsted, Twill, Solid, Slight sheen, Raw silk, Tweed (tightly woven), Houndstooth or strong check, Linen, Bold plaid, Suede (peaked lapel, stiff interfacing), Denim.

☐ **Pants**

  Style: Plain front, Pleated, Cuffs, if you're 6' or over.

  Fabric: Tightly woven, Smooth Texture, Gabardine, Worsted.

☐ **Sweaters**

  Style: Turtlenecks, V-necks.

  Designs: Geometric, Stripes, Blocks, Aztec designs, Abstracts, Solids.

☐ **Sport Shirts**

  Style: No collar, Nehru, Straight silhouette, Polo, V-neck.

  Fabric: Crisp fabrics, Solid, Stripes, Checks.

☐ **Shoes**

  European loafer, Gucci loafer, Boat shoe.

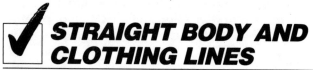 # *STRAIGHT BODY AND CLOTHING LINES*

☐ **Face Shape:**

  Square, Rectangular.

☐ **Body Shape:**

  Rectangular, Square.

☐ **Overall Impression:**

  Rectangular, Straight Lines.

☐ **Bone Structure - Body Proportions:**

  Small 5'9'' or under, Average 5'10'' to 6'1'', Large 6'2'' or over.

YOUR BUSINESS LOOK

- Suits:

  Style: European cut (padded shoulders, waist emphasis), Updated American, Single-breasted, Double-breasted, Notched lapel.

  Fabric: Moderate to tightly woven, Worsted, Sharkskin, Pin stripe: 1/8" - 1/4" - 1/2", Herringbone, Linen, Silk, Glenn plaid, Flannel, Cashmere, Gabardine, Crisp poplin.

- Dress Shirts

  Style: Tapered fit, Pin collar, Tab collar, Standard collar, Contrasting collar and cuffs.

  Fabric: Broadcloth, Oxfordcloth, Stripe, Pin stripe, Pin point, Check, Solid.

- Ties

  Designs: Solid, Club, Stripe, Foulard, Polka dot (pin), Crisp paisley.

  Fabric: Matte finish, Silk, Raw silk.

- Shoes

  Tie, Plain slip-on, Thin sole.

- Top Coat

  Style: Fly front, Trench, Single-breasted, Double-breasted.

  Fabric: Cashmere, Tweed, Herringbone, Twill.

YOUR CASUAL LOOK

- Sport Coat

  Style: Updated American, Single-breasted, Double-breasted, Notched lapel, Top-stiching.

  Fabric: Cahsmere, Cashmere blend, Flannel, Linen, Herringbone, Houndstooth check, Suede (stiff interfacing).

- Pants

  Style: Pleated, Plain front, Cuffs, if 6' or over.

  Fabric: Wool flannel, Worsted, Poplin, Linen, Moderate to crisp fabrics, Crisp fabrics, Denim, Gabardine.

- Sweaters

  Style: Turtleneck, Crew neck, V-neck.

  Designs: Plaids, Blocks, Solids.

- Sport Shirts

Style: Button-down collar, Standard collar, No collar, Polo.
Fabric: Broadcloth, Oxfordcloth, Crisp fabrics, Checks, Plaids, Solids.
- Shoes
Boat shoe, Tassel loafer, Oxford loafer, Gucci loafer.

CONTOURED BODY AND CLOTHING LINES

☐ **Face Shape:**
Oval, Round, Oblong.
☐ **Body Shape:**
Rectangular (softened edges), Ellipse.
☐ **Overall Impressions:**
Elliptical, Contoured Lines.
☐ **Body Proportions:**
Small 5'9'' or under, Average 5'10'' to 6'1'', Large 6'2'' or over.

YOUR BUSINESS LOOK

- Suits
Style: Ivy League cut, Updated American, Single-breasted, Notched lapel.
Fabric: Soft texture, Worsted, Wool flannel, Nubby texture, Cashmere, Dull finish, Herringbone, Glenn Plaid (flannel), Chalk stripe 1/8'' - 1/4'' - 1/2'', Tweed.
- Dress Shirts
Style: Full cut, Medium range fit, Button-down collar, Standard collar, Tab collar.
Fabric: Oxfordcloth, Broadcloth, Oxford stripe, Solid, End-on-End.
- Ties
Designs: Solid, Stripe, Club, Foulard, Paisley.
Fabric: Matte finish, Silk, Wool, Knit.
- Shoes
Tie, Plain slip-on, Wing tip.

- Top Coat
  Style: Raglan sleeve, Fly front, Single-breasted.
  Fabric: Cashmere, Wool flannel, Tweed, Herringbone.

YOUR CASUAL LOOK

- Sport Coat
  Style: Single-breasted, Notched lapel, Curved lapel, Top-stitching, Ivy League cut.
  Fabric: Dull finish, Flannel, Suede, Cashmere, Corduroy, Hopsack, Herringbone, Nubby fabric, Tweed, Plaid.
- Pants
  Style: Plain front, Pleated front, Elasticized waist, Cuffs, if you're 6' or over.
  Fabric: Soft fabric, Wool flannel, Corduroy, Soft denim, Ribbed, Worsted.
- Sweaters
  Style: Crew neck, Cardigan, V-neck (very soft fabric).
  Designs: Tweeds, Paisleys, Plaids, Blended stripes, Solids, Heather, Cashmere (or blend).
- Sport Shirts
  Style: Soft neckline, Button-down collar, No collar, Polo.
  Fabric: Plaid, Tattersall, Knits, Solids.
- Shoes
  Boat shoe, Gucci loafer, Tassel loafer, Penny loafer.

LEARN TO IDENTIFY THE STYLES OF YOUR BEST CASUAL LOOKS

Sharp-Straight Body Types	Straight Body Types	Contoured Body Types

When choosing items for your casual wardrobe, apply the same *Successful Style* concepts that work when choosing a suit: the cut of the garment should be a reflection of your body's shape.

Applying this concept and knowing what to look for will reduce the time you need to shop. More importantly you'll find the clothes will work together when you get them home.

A Few Tips on Going Casual

Shipping magnate Aristotle Onassis felt "casual" no matter what he was wearing.

"Know what's right at the right time," he said. The rest of it is relatively easy.

The listings earlier on showed you what looks best for your body shape. You can almost play it by the "numbers" and look good. What you need is to develop the Onassian nose for knowing what's right and when. It certainly pays off at work, and it's critical to off-hours as well.

If you think about it, dressing for the office isn't nearly as demanding as what to wear outside the office. At work you've got your "corporate uniform." But if one of your best clients invites you to his house for a barbeque, what do you wear?

You can always ask a colleague who has been to the house what the others are wearing. Chances are he (or she) will say that people wore whatever they were comfortable in. Some men wore sport coats with ties, loosened at the collar; others had no ties. Some wore no jacket, one or two were in designer jeans. The client wore an old shirt and shoes and a charcoal-stained apron with bold lettering that declared, "I'M THE CHEF AROUND HERE!"

He was comfortable, and the others were, too.

Most of the men we've done business with have agreed on certain ground rules for casual dressing. Here's their concensus:

- If the occasion is indoors, wear a jacket.
- A necktie is unnecessary in any casual setting. You may wear one if you wish, so long as it, too, is as casual as your jacket and slacks. The tie you won't wear to the office because it's too colorful will probably work.
- Wear easy shoes. No wingtips. Mocs are fine. Clean boat shoes are fine if they go with what you're wearing. A very well-known woman novelist (and former columnist on men) swore that, in her Manhattan circles, any man who didn't settle for Bass Weejun loafers was probably giving the matter too much thought!

Outdoor Casual

- If the occasion is outdoors, jackets and open collars are the norm. Slacks that are light and comfortable are important. You'll be on your feet a lot, so give yourself some space with loose trousers.

- Dark shades are okay, but out in the open a mixture of natural earth tones and a dash of color make it a brighter day. It's nice to shine a bit.

- If you don't wear the usual jacket, maybe a bush jacket from the Banana Republic will do. (Only in Key West is a bush jacket considered more-or-less formal.)

- *Sans* jacket, good quality polo shirts are fine. A madras shirt is okay. Still, most men feel more at ease with a jacket of some kind. After all, if you need it, you've got it. If you don't, you can always put it in the trunk of your car.

- Beware of athletic outfits. Unless you know the guests and your host and hostess very well, don't risk doing an imitation of a Boston Marathoner — unless you've actually come in among the top three runners. You'll find that, in practice, even famous jocks opt for a jacket or a nice shirt, slacks, and an easygoing shoes.

- If you're wearing a good silk jacket and the client who has invited you to the bash wants you to help him slop on the barbeque sauce, *take off the jacket!* He's inviting you into his "kitchen," so roll up your sleeves and dig in.

- What to wear on a boat is a book in itself. It all comes down to dressing as you would for an outdoor gathering. But there is one hard and fast rule: *always wear soft-soled shoes:* Sperry Docksiders, rubber-soled mocs, running shoes. It helps you keep your balance on deck and the soles won't scuff that expensive teak wood. Don't wear a skipper's cap unless you actually are one.

- Leather patches, tweeds, brass — all these touches work outdoors.

- If you have a jacket with a club emblem, casual is the place for you to wear it.

- Stick to the casual clothing you're most comfortable with. In Florida, casual may be close to being half-naked. In Maine, it's overalls and work boots. In California, it's "Hollywood." In Texas, it's riding boots and 10-gallon hats. Don't try to regionalize yourself unless you are very familiar with a region's idiosyncracies.

- Enjoy yourself! No matter what you're wearing, once you're on the scene, pitch in and have a good time. Attitude will overcome all if the clothing complements you, expresses your personality, and is appropriate for the time and place.

Shopping Guidelines

- Go with a Plan.
- Use your priority shopping list and avoid impulse buying.
- Know Where and When.
- Shop twice a year. Shop in August/September for Fall/Winter. Shop in April/May for Spring/Summer. Shop in a store or stores that carry a full range of wardrobe prices. Look for the clothes that fit your personal sytle.
- Know How To Spend.
- When buying a suit, the most important item in your wardrobe, get the best quality within your price range. Before you make a purchase, try an expensive suit to get an idea on how it feels, how it looks, watch the fabric, the tailoring, the details. When trying on a similar suit, the quality of the fabric and the fit should be your main consideration.
- When updating your wardrobe to complement your coloring and body lines, purchase a few shirts and ties that are right for you and will make a suit work better until you can replace it.
- Beware of "special purchase" items. Sometimes they may be below the store's usual quality.
- When buying the sale items, check the quality of the garment. They may be off-season. Be sure they are not off-style.
- When buying accessories do not compromise in quality; they make or break your look.
- When buying a suit wear a shirt and the shoes that you usually wear. Try the pants and jacket with the items you regularly carry such as billfold, cardholder, etc.
- Buy a suit and at least 3 shirts and 3 ties that will go with it.

✓ GETTING IT ALTOGETHER CHECKLIST

Since our contoured, straight, and sharp-straight charts sum up the essentials of this chapter, we'll present a few "finishing touches" to back them up. They should prove quite useful in getting it all together.

☐ No matter what your shape may be, and no matter how well the charts work for you, it's up to you to personalize your style. Using different fabrics, colors, and accessories in a distinctive way will give an outfit your special logo.

☐ Body shape can and does change over time. Your trusty bathroom scale, a tape measure, and your existing wardrobe fit are the barometers of change. Use them often. Adjust as required.

☐ Office and casual wardrobes shouldn't be mixed. Build each on a separate foundation.

☐ There's a difference between indoor and outdoor casual. The first is usually a little more formal than the latter. In either case, comfort, fit, and an "easy" look are paramount.

☐ Avoid imitating celebrities. Remember they are dressed in what amounts to a costume whenever you see them. There's always an element of exaggeration in the way they look — an exaggeration that works beautifully on the screen or on the tube. In real life, however, *understatement* and *quiet good taste* are key to looking great.

☐ At work or at play, avoid wearing any single item that draws attention away from the rest of you. You want others to focus on you and what you have to say, not some extravagant designer's idea of chic.

☐ Experiment with the fabrics and other details listed in the charts presented earlier. Confine your experiments to the mirror at the menswear store; don't spring them on an unsuspecting world at great personal cost and/or embarrassment.

☐ Many men depend at some extent on the women in their lives to help them make clothing selections. That's okay, up to a point. Women aren't any better than men in this department, only more experienced. However, their experience is often in the area of women's clothing. They too need to learn the rules of the road of men's dressing. Work to be your own best judge of what's right for you.

☐ Casual occasions give you a chance to use accents and accessories you normally wouldn't bring to the office. Ascots, club ties, blazers with emblems, arty belt buckles — all are designed for the easy life. Make tasteful and judicious use of them to brighten your image and add a bit of sparkle to the scene.

☐ Men's magazines are notorious for advertising wardrobes best suited to younger men. Don't add fuel to the fire of a mid- life crisis by imitating advertisements designed for bodies and minds half your age. And if you're not middle-aged, don't be seduced by what *Gentleman's Quarterly* swears is the latest and hippest. You are neither a clothes horse nor a walking billboard of labels.

☐ Quality is the first and last court of resort in making the right selections. Think "investment" whenever you purchase something for your wardrobe.

☐ Smooth over body flaws with great fit — not color or trendy designs.

☐ It's always best to wear a jacket to casual affairs. If you need it, you've got it. If it's out of place, hide it until you leave. Make sure the jacket is high quality but not the serious business item you'd wear to work. Relax! You're there to have fun.

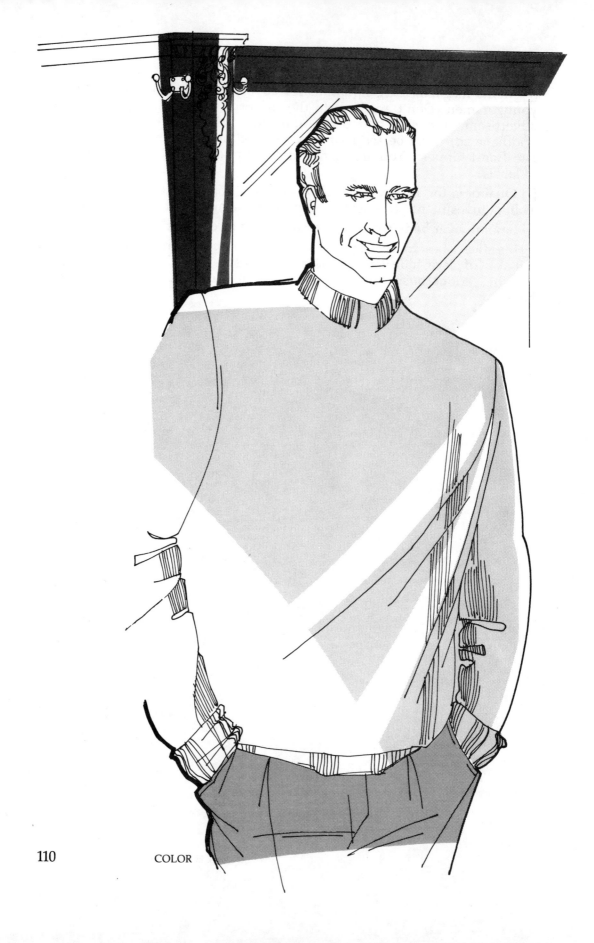

110   COLOR

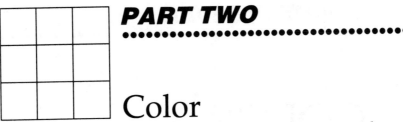

PART TWO

Color

Wearing the right colors is an art and a science, both of which are easy and exciting to master.

The first thing to understand is that color, like clothing lines and styles, needs to be individualized, it has to be as personal a choice as selecting the right cut and fabric for your particular body shape. The same four rules apply that have been generalized in the description of the well-dressed man.

Colors must complement you physically, express your personality, must be appropriate for the occasion, and the use and combinations must be current.

It would be wonderful if we could simply wear the colors that appeal to us the most. You can do that, of course, if you're one of those lucky people with a flawlessly innate sense of what works and what doesn't. But for most of us it's a matter of learning the rules, and that's what this section is all about.Color — one of the most critically important elements of personal style — is the first order of business in this section on Successful Style.

Because color is probably the most subjective and least understood facet of dress, we've reduced (if not eliminated) the guesswork with a simple, easy-to-follow series of charts. Once you discover which color chart describes you best, you'll always be able to make the correct picks, and mixing and matching will help expand your present wardrobe.

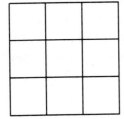

CHAPTER SEVEN

COLOR AT WORK

How To Make It Work For You

Wearing the right colors can brighten your whole appearance. It can create mood, dash, individuality — even power. Dark colors, for example, project strength and authority. Have you ever noticed that many successful attorneys plead their cases in a dark suit, crisp white shirt, and a sober-looking necktie? They dress this way for affect — and it works! On the other hand, someone who wants to affect a light, breezy feeling will wear a tan or light gray suit, a pastel shirt, and tie with more color. The lighter and brighter colors lessen one's presence and diminish the hard edges.

All of this occurs in the eye of the beholder; it's totally subjective, neither positive nor negative. It is true that there is a general consensus of opinion on the psychological aspects of color and their effects in general. These are the facts we are working with along with our own professional opinions. But think for a moment: As an attorney defending a client facing a serious charge, which colors would you choose for the courtroom? Dark, of course, as we mentioned above. Just how dark to maintain the appearance of power, your power, and not the color overpowering you, will be discussed in the next section. It will of course depend on your personal color characteristics as your clothing line selection depends on your face and body shape.

The choice of the courtroom suit will not affect the cause of justice, except that the judge and the jurors will be more inclined to notice you and pay slightly closer attention to your words, if you are presenting a powerful look without being overpowering.

Strictly for Looks

We'll return to the "power" aspects of color later in this chapter. For now, let's concentrate on the ways color can make you look terrific all the time.

Wearing the right colors *enhances your complexion.* Lines and wrinkles seem to disappear; circles under the eyes are less apparent; you take on a visible "glow." This can often be seen with renewed color in the cheeks and skintone. The "five o'clock shadow", will often seem less obvious since complementary colors cause less shadowing on the face.

The end product of such enhancement creates a younger, more relaxed appearance. If you are young anyway, you'll simply look as if you've put in a few overtime sessions at the health club.

The right colors also enhance your eyes. Women learned this trick (it's one of their wiles) on the first sunrise of the first morning of recorded history. It's about time men learned it too. Proper color combinations make your eyes brighter, more attentive-looking. Eye contact, as important in business as in the bedroom, is noticeably magnified when your colors are right. You gain credibility and trust. Complementary colors add harmony and balance to your appearance and invest real value in what you're wearing. If your $1000 Armani suit clashes with your skintone, hair, and eyes, you may as well polish your car with it.

The bottom line is this. Color is the final, and perhaps most visible, element of looking good. It's the finishing all-important touch that makes the line and scale work.

The Power Factor and More

Color conveys power. It can also convey other messages.

If you're not entirely convinced by the example of the attorney in the courtroom, think about how color is shrewdly used in product development.

Start in your own kitchen. Your refrigerator and most appliances are white or pale shades of other colors. The idea is to convey the notion of clean spic-and-span orderliness. This has been the message that was crucial up until a few years ago. As gourmet cooking became more popular, many switched to stainless steel, the professional look used in restaurant kitchens by professional cooks.

Just as colors help change the mood of the room, they create an indication of the type of use expected in that room and very importantly set a date — how current, how new, how fashionable, what era, much the same way our styles of clothes project a date. With color — like line, detail, and style in general, we must update or the message sent to others says, "I'm behind."

There are many products that are less affected by current changes in fashion trends but their success still depends on hidden messages in the packages. Your Braun electric razor is probably a flat gun-metal blue. The typical all-male hi-tech hue says power, reliability, function.

Out on the street you'll notice that your local policeman's uniform is either paramilitary brown, blue, or flat black. These shades say law and order, authority, raw power. Ask yourself how seriously you would take a policeman in an all-white uniform in New York City. The answer is, not very! Naval officers wear "dress whites," but at sea the military hues are the order of the day and that means dark or khaki colors. In other parts of the world, especially tropical countries, white may be used for climate and/or cultural reasons. Any cultural use of color has its own built-in message, more strong than any that is learned indirectly.

The same messages apply in the corporate world. Navy and gray are the classic order of the day. These are the conservative uniforms of business worldwide — universal colors of the banners under which deals are made and positions decided. These are the colors you'll wear when you go before the Securities and Exchange Commission examiners who must decide if your company may trade on the Big Board. Surely you won't present yourself in a white suit and flower tie — not when the stakes are high.

In summary, dark colors convey the message of authority, power, and confidence. Therefore, they should be used for more formal situations or when you need to exert power and authority. Medium colors are better used for staff meetings and days when a more casual or friendly atmosphere is desired.

Neutrals form the foundation of your wardrobe, especially in suits. Neutrals can be worn with all other colors, are conservative and those you are least likely to tire of. They have the least cultural and psychological effect and are, therefore, safe.

Bright colors should be used in accents to complement a bold look. They should be used in small amounts in ties, pocket scarves, etc.

Contrasting colors should be used for definition. The more contrast, the more powerful the look.

No one quite understands why these rules work the way they do. There is little historical evidence that navy and gray have been the immortal shades of commerce. The ancient Greeks and Romans wore light colors exclusively until they discovered certain dies, taken from sea snails, that gave them "royal" purples. The purple was rare and therefore reserved for the ruling class. It can be argued and debated that this is the real origin of today's obsession with blues and grays. It's really academic. What counts is that, for whatever reason, men are expected to do serious business in serious colors.

Just as navy and gray suits are a necessary and important part of your corporate color wardrobe, there's another color rule you should know. It has to do with raincoats, and it's just the opposite of the standard suit colorations. Beige or tan are, for reasons that may not be quite tangible, considered more credible and professional. They project a more solid, classic look than black, navy or dark brown. Some fashion designers believe that beige and tan outerwear is preferred because it doesn't clash with the navy and gray you're wearing underneath. In England, where this rule seems etched in marble, the idea is that one doesn't reveal oneself or one's true status on the street.

It is also important to note as we shall see in the following section that because of the elements in our skintone, hair, and eye color, various shades of warm beige and gray-beige are complementary to everyone's coloring.

Does all this seem either antiquated or confusing? Well maybe so. What *isn't* antique is that bucking convention with clothing — be it via color or cut — makes getting to the top and/or staying there just that much harder. Learning and playing by the rules can be easy. They are not so rigid that you do not have personal freedom and choices. They are merely guidelines that will give you the extra edge and guarantee you the confidence necessary for success. (At the end of this chapter you'll find the charts to help you select shirts and ties to go with your navy and gray to assure personalization).

Undertones, Depth, and Brightness

Before we delve into specific guidelines to help you to select your correct wardrobe of colors, it is important to discuss the basic characteristics of color and how they compare with the color of your hair, eyes, and skin.

One of the easiest ways to describe color is to go with what is immediately apparent: apples are red, carrots are orange, snow is white, skies are blue. You might consider these simple descriptions as "level one" of color identification. But it is important to consider two other characteristics; depth and brightness.

Undertones-Below the Surface: Undertones are the yellows or blues that are added to colors to make them "warm" or "cool." They are not always instantly visible. If you've ever added colors to house paint, for instance, adding a touch of yellow to blue you get aquamarine, a more yellow-based color. The yellow- or gold-based colors are called warm colors, the more blue-based are called cool. For simplicity we will consider warm and cool colors to account for the undertone.

Consider an orange-red or blue-red. The orange-red has a yellow base, the blue-red a blue base. A great many colors are combinations of undertones with almost equal amounts of yellow and blue. These are called true colors. Consider an orange-red, true red, and blue-red.

Light and Shade Equals Depth: The second characteristic of color is "depth" — how dark or light a particular color may be. Consider a color from its darkest shade to its lightest — from black to white with various shades of gray in between. A deep red or maroon, for example, runs the spectrum all the way to pale pink. The steps in between represent the level of depth. We will consider deep and light colors. Deep ranging from dark to medium and light from medium to pale. Obviously there are colors in the medium range that take a judgment call as to whether they are more light or more dark.

Brightness: Still another important characteristic is "brightness." This refers to how vivid or muted a color may be. Muted colors have been softened by adding gray to the color to lessen its intensity. Going from a brilliant fire engine red to a pink blush is an example of how colors are toned down, or muted. In our third color characteristic we will consider muted and bright as definition of intensity.

Personal Coloring

Your personal coloring has the same three characteristics: an undertone, depth, and level of brightness. Your personal coloring is determined by your skintone, hair, and the color of your eyes. In the same way that the cut of your clothes complements your body lines, the colors you wear do the same thing.

We can wear all kinds of colors, but it's the undertone, depth, and intensity that are important. What you're after is balance and harmony so that the colors are a natural extension of you. By wearing colors that have the same or similar characteristics as your coloring, balance will result. There are some colors that you wear that may not be perfectly harmonious. They can be combined with other colors to make the total balance. Given the general guidelines for colors in business, it is necessary to understand how to efficiently use those combinations. The bottom line is that color must complement you physically, express your personality, be appropriate for the occasion, and current.

The basic elements of natural coloration focus on your skin tone, along with the color of our hair and eyes. Taken together they project colorations that can be described as warm, cool, light, deep, muted, or bright.

Let's start with skin. Skintone is determined by melanin, carotin, and hemoglobin.

Melanin is a dark pigment found in the skin, the retina, and human hair. It is often described as brown to orange-red in color. Carotin (sometimes spelled Carotene) is an orange-yellow, reddish compound occurring as a pigment in humans and plants. It is often a color that appears on the skin's surface and can be affected by diet, drugs, etc. Hemoglobin is the oxygen-bearing protein in red blood cells and is red in coloration.

Depending on the amounts of each of these elements in our bodies, our coloring will appear to be either more warm or more cool, light or deep, bright or muted.

No one is all cool since the elements in our skintones are predominantly warm. However, to the human eye, some people will appear more warm or golden than others. Some will have a distribution that makes the skintone appear neutral. Others will appear cool, pinky, or rosy. It is important to look at your overall coloring and determine which characteristic is most dominant. What do you see first when looking at yourself in the mirror? What color is your hair? Eyes? Is your skin pink, beige, or golden?

By determining your most dominant color characteristic you will be able to select your best colors — those that complement you physically. Once you understand your complementary colors, you will understand how dark your navy and gray should be, what color shirts and ties to wear, and how to select your casual colors.

Which Best Describes Your Coloring?

Warm: The "warm" person projects a total golden glow. There will be evidence of true golden undertones in the hair, eyes, and skintone. Hair will be red, auburn, golden blonde, yellow brown or strawberry. You may in fact have been called a redhead at some point. Eye color will be hazel, green, teal, brown, or topaz. A ruddy earthtone will be projected in the eye color with gold or green combinations. Warm skintone is bronze, golden beige, ivory, and often has freckles. In general, warm coloring will be medium in depth, not too light or dark.

If you can describe your coloring as "warm" you will always be successful wearing warm-based colors of medium depth. *See examples and charts.*

Warm

☐ **Colors-Warm**
- **Suggested:** ivory, beige, golden browns, camel, medium gray (for business), medium navy (for business), peach, teal and periwinkle, warm reds, warm greens, rust, mahogany, turquoise, gold.
- **Avoid:** pure white (may be used for a shirt color), black, pink, burgundy, bright blues, blue-reds.

☐ **Suggested Shirt and Tie Combinations-Warm**
- **Navy Suit:** medium navy, avoid dark shades.
- **Gray suit:** medium gray, avoid blue-gray or charcoal.
- **Shirts:** white, blue, soft white, buff, ivory, beige, light yellow, peach.
- **Ties:** tomato red, bittersweet, rust, mahogany, teal, gold, golden tan, yellow, gray, navy.

Cool: A "cool" person often has a rose or pink complexion. It is often described as rosy or dusty. Don't confuse this with peach coloring or a high red color. "Cool" coloring in general will be in the mid-tone range, not too dark or light.

Hair color will be ash brown, dark brown, or deep ash blonde. There may be some warm highlights but they will not be obvious or easily seen. Overall an ash color will be projected. Remember, everyone's hair has some red highlights. In the cool person these are subtle. As our hair grays it loses pigment and becomes more ash-colored. Our appearance often softens.

Skintone will be beige, rose-beige, pink, taupe, and will often project a blue or gray undertone. Eye color will be blue-gray, gray-blue, or cool green. If brown, it will be rosy or gray-brown.

If your coloring can be described as cool you can successfully wear cool-based colors that are neither too dark nor too light. *See examples and charts.*

Cool

☐ **Colors-Cool**
- **Suggested:** gray, navy cocoa, taupe, soft white, blue-red, any blue, blue-greens, pinks, purples, plums, lavenders, burgundy.
- **Avoid:** golden browns, yellow-greens, peach, ivory, warm reds, camels, beige, warm turquoise, orange.

☐ **Suggested Shirt and Tie Combinations-Cool**
- **Navy suit:** — avoid darkest shades.
- **Gray suit:** blue-gray, medium gray, charcoal gray.
- **Shirts:** white, light blue, soft white, light pink, icy gray, icy aqua, icy lavender.
- **Ties:** blue-red, burgundy, navy, gray, plum, gray-blue, yellow.

Deep: The "deep" characteristic is the easiest to see. Do you have dark hair and eyes? If so, you're deep. How deep? Haircolor will range from black to deep brown, from a chestnut or Auburn color to blue-black. Eyes will also be deep — dark brown, brown-black, deep hazel, or dark olive.

Skintone will generally be a beige color, however may be olive, or bronze. There are warm and cool undertones in the deep person. If you are deep you can successfully wear deep colors that are not too blue or too gold. *See examples and charts.*

Deep

☐ **Colors-Deep**
- **Suggested:** white, soft white, charcoal gray, black, taupe, true red, mahogany, teal, pine green, true green, turquoise, true blues, yellow.
- **Avoid:** light colors, pastel colors, plum, blue-reds, oranges.

☐ **Suggested Shirt and Tie Combinations-Deep**
- **Navy Suit:** medium to dark.
- **Gray Suit:** medium to charcoal.
- **Shirts:** white, icy blue, soft white, icy aqua, icy yellow, icy gray.
- **Ties:** true red, mahogany, lemon yellow, navy, gray, teal, yellow.

Light: If your coloring can be described as light, your hair color will be blonde — golden or ash — medium to dark. Your hair may darken when not exposed to sunlight and then rapidly lighten as bleached by the sun. Skintone will be medium to light and may appear peach or rosy. There will be little contrast between hair color and skintone. Eye color will be gray, blue, green, or a combination. Eye color will appear to change colors from blue to gray to green. It will not be brown, deep hazel, or deep blue. *See examples and charts.*

Light

☐ **Colors-Light**
- **Suggested:** soft white, rose beige, medium navy (business), medium gray (business), cocoa, camel, watermelon red, medium blues, coral pinks, pinks, periwinkle blues, glue-greens.
- **Avoid:** pure white (may be used for a shirt color), dark colors, black, charcoal gray, blue-reds, plums, oranges.

☐ **Suggested Shirt and Tie Combinations-Light**
- **Navy Suit:** medium navy, avoid dark shades.
- **Gray Suit:** light to medium, blue gray, avoid charcoal gray.
- **Shirts:** white, light blue, soft white, rose-beige, warm pink, light yellow, buff, light gray.
- **Ties:** watermelon red, navy, gray, yellow, turquoise, blue.

Muted: When we refer to muted colors, we are talking about colors that have been "toned down" by adding gray to soften, or "knock off" the edge of a color. Interestingly enough, grayed down or muted colors have a weightiness or richness about them that produces a less delicate look than light colors without getting dark.

Muted coloring has strength but not depth. Hair color will be light, ash blonde, ash brown, or medium blonde. Skintone will range from golden to beige to ivory, often with an absence of any cheek color. With the light hair, eyes may be brown, hazel, teal. The main difference between the muted and light will be the eye color that projects richness to the overall coloring — hazel, teal, turquoise, etc. The coloring range will not be light or dark but medium in depth. There will in fact be a balance with a "no color" look. If your coloring can be described as muted you will successfully wear softened colors of medium intensity. *See examples and charts.*

Muted

☐ **Colors-Muted**
  - **Suggested:** soft white, oyster white, beige, blue-gray (for business), medium navy (business), medium rose or cocoa brown, blue-green, grayed green, tomato red, coral, warm pink, periwinkle, teal, mahogany, medium blues.
  - **Avoid:** bright colors, high contrast, blue-reds, orange, golden browns.

☐ **Suggested Shirt and Tie Combinations-Muted**
  - **Navy Suit:** grayed navy, avoid dark navy.
  - **Gray Suit:** medium blue-gray, soft charcoal.
  - **Shirts:** white, soft white, light blue, rose-beige, warm pink, light aqua, buff, light gray.
  - **Ties:** tomato red, bittersweet, teal, mahogany, navy, gray, yellow, rust.

Bright: The "bright" person has a crisp, clear look derived from a strong contrast between skin and hair color and the jewel-like clarity of the eye color. There are two types of coloring that can be called "bright."

The first is the person whose hair color contrasts sharply with the skintone. Hair color will be dark brown, sometimes even black, or ash brown. Skin color will be almost transparent —ivory or porcelain. Accompanying this contrast in skin and hair color will be bright, clear eye color in jewel tones — blue, green, turquoise, or violet. They will not be dark brown. This type of bright person has often been confused with the "deep."

The brightness of the eyes alone will demand a balance of clarity that is lost with colors that are too deep.

Others who can be described as having bright coloring but do not have as much contrast in the hair and skintone include those whose eye color is true and jewel-like, blue, green, turquoise, etc. Skintone will be a bit more golden and hair not as deep; eyebrows and lashes will be dark. If your coloring can be described as bright you can successfully wear colors that are clear — primary colors — that are neither too deep nor too light. *See examples and charts.*

Bright

☐ **Colors-Bright**
- **Suggested:** navy, gray, white, soft white, taupe, true red, true green, true blue, bright pink, coral pink, turquoise, choose colors that create some contrast.
- **Avoid:** deep colors, muted colors, camel, warm browns, blue-reds, orange.

☐ **Suggested Shirt and Tie Combinations-Bright**
- **Navy Suit:** medium to dark, avoid muted navy.
- **Gray Suit:** medium to charcoal.
- **Shirts:** white, soft white, light blue, soft white, warm pink, icy aqua, icy gray.
- **Ties:** true red, clear navy, gray, lemon yellow, turquoise, blue.

Color Anyone Can Wear

Universal colors are colors that can be successfully worn by everyone since they are neither too dark or too light, wram or cool, muted or bright.

- Soft white
- Buff
- Coral pink
- Turquoise
- Periwinkle blue
- Blue-green
- Taupe
- True gray
- Watermelon
- Teal
- Greyed navy
- Medium violet

Caucasian Color Characteristics

☐ **Warm**
- **General Impression:** total golden glow, medium depth, medium intensity.
- **Hair:** golden brown, chestnut, auburn, gold, red, strawberry, blonde highlights.
- **Eyes:** green, hazel, turquoise, topaz, teal, not light blue or gray-blue.
- **Skin:** golden beige, ivory, bronze, freckles.

☐ **Cool**
- **General Impression:** ash, rosy, pink, soft, medium depth, medium intensity.
- **Hair:** ash brown, dark brown, deep blonde.
- **Eyes:** rose-brown, gray-brown, blue, blue-green, grayed blue, not hazel or green.
- **Skin:** pink, rose-beige, beige, sometimes sallow.

☐ **Deep**
- **General Impression:** evidence of both warm and cool undertones, strong-contrast-vivid, medium intensity.
- **Hair:** dark brown, chestnut, auburn, black, brown-black.
- **Eyes:** dark brown, rose-brown, deep hazel, deep green.
- **Skin:** olive, bronze, beige, maybe sallow.

☐ **Light**
- **General Impression:** evidence of warm and cool undertones, soft, delicate, fair — little contrast, between hair and skin, medium intensity.
- **Hair:** most often blonde (light to medium), ash brown or light brown possible.
- **Eyes:** blue, blue-green, aqua, not deep, hazel, or brown.
- **Skin:** ivory, pink, peach, soft beige.

☐ **Bright**
- **General Impression:** evidence of warm and cool undertones, contrasting hair and skin color, crisp, clear, high intensity.
- **Hair:** medium to dark brown, ash-golden brown, black.
- **Eyes:** blue-green, steel gray, turquoise, deep blue, not dark.
- **Skin:** ivory, porcelain, beige, translucent, sometimes ruddy.

☐ **Muted**
- **General Impression:** evidence of warm, and cool undertones, medium depth, dusty, soft, low intensity.
- **Hair:** ash brown, ash blonde, deep golden blonde, golden browns.
- **Eyes:** hazel — most common, medium-dark brown, green, teal, not light or gray blue.
- **Skin:** ivory, beige, bronze, absence of color, opaque, freckles.

Black Color Characteristics

☐ **Warm**
- **General Impression:** total golden glow, medium depth, medium intensity.
- **Hair:** brown, golden brown, brown-black, chestnut.
- **Eyes:** warm brown, topaz, deep brown, hazel.
- **Skin:** bronze, caramel, mahogany, golden brown, light golden brown, freckles.

☐ **Cool**
- **General Impression:** ash, gray, rosy, medium depth, medium intensity.
- **Hair:** black, ash brown, blue-black.
- **Eyes:** brown-black, black, gray-brown, rose-brown.
- **Skin:** rose-brown, gray-brown, cocoa, dark brown, soft blue-black.

☐ **Deep**
- **General Impression:** evidence of warm and cool undertones, strong contrast, vivid, medium intensity.
- **Hair:** black, blue-black, brown-black.
- **Eyes:** black, brown-black, red-brown, brown.
- **Skin:** blue-black, deep brown, rose-brown, mahogany, bronze.

☐ **Light**
- **General Impression:** evidence of warm and cool undertones, soft, delicate, less contrast between hair and skin, medium intensity.
- **Hair:** soft black, brown-black, brown, light brown, red-brown, ash brown.
- **Eyes:** soft black, brown, rose-brown.
- **Skin:** light brown, caramel, bronze, rose-beige, deep beige, cocoa.

☐ **Brights**
- **General Impression:** evidence of warm and cool undertones, contrast in color of skin and hair, bright, clear, and high intensity.
- **Hair:** black, brown-black, ash brown, deep brown.
- **Eyes:** black, brown-black.
- **Skin:** light brown, deep beige, cocoa, caramel.

☐ **Muted**
- **General Impression:** evidence of warm and cool undertones, medium in depth, soft, dusty-low intensity.
- **Hair:** brown, ash brown, brown-black.
- **Eyes:** brown-black, black, gray-brown, hazel, rose-brown.
- **Skin:** light brown, cocoa, rose-brown, beige, opaque, freckles, absence of strong color.

Asian Color Characteristics

☐ **Warm**
- **General Impression:** total golden glow, medium depth, medium intensity.
- **Hair:** golden brown, auburn, dark brown, chestnut.
- **Eyes:** warm brown, brown-black, hazel, deep brown, topaz.
- **Skin:** golden beige, ivory, bronze, freckles.

☐ **Cool**
- **General Impression:** ash, rosy, pink, medium depth, medium intensity.
- **Hair:** blue-black, black, brown-black, chestnut, dark brown.
- **Eyes:** black, gray-brown, rose-brown.
- **Skin:** rose-beige, gray-beige, pink, sometimes sallow.

☐ **Deep**
- **General Impression:** evidence of warm and cool undertones, strong, contrast, vivid, medium intensity.
- **Hair:** blue-black, black, brown-black, chestnut, dark brown.
- **Eyes:** Black, brown-black, red-brown.
- **Skin:** olive, bronze, beige.

☐ **Light**
- **General Impression:** evidence of warm and cool undertones, soft, delicate, contrast between hair and skintone, medium intensity.
- **Hair:** brown-black, ash brown, brown, soft black.
- **Eyes:** red-brown, brown-black, black, gray-black.
- **Skin:** rose-beige, ivory, pink, beige, pale.

☐ **Bright**
- **General Impression:** evidence of warm and cool undertones, contrast in color of hair and skintone, contrast between hair and skintone; light skin — dark hair, bright, translucent, high intensity.
- **Hair:** black, brown-black, dark brown.
- **Eyes:** black, brown-black.
- **Skin:** ivory, porcelain.

☐ **Muted**
- **General Impression:** evidence of warm and cool undertones, medium in depth, soft, dusty, low intensity.
- **Hair:** brown, mahogany, ash brown, soft black.
- **Eyes:** brown, rose-brown, hazel, brown-black, gray-brown.
- **Skin:** beige, red-beige, bronze, absence of color — opaque, freckles, opaque.

Colors For All Occasions

Now that you have identified your coloring, you can select those that are the most complementary to you. Notice that these recommendations include colors for all occasions. It is important to remember that not all of these colors are correct for the corporate look. Just as there is a need for different types of clothes for different occasions, there are certain colors that are more casual, more formal, or more corporate.

Neutral colors (gray, beige, navy, camel, brown) are more conservative and classical. These should be the mainstay of your wardrobe, especially your suits. The grays and navys are critical colors for your corporate wardrobe.

Personalizing Navy and Gray

Those with golden coloring need to wear shirt and tie combinations that relate specifically to their golden-base coloring since most navy and gray suits are not considered "warm." Browns and tans will be complementary but must be used with care in corporate settings.

Those with "light" coloring must be careful to select shirt and tie combinations that create enough contrast for a corporate power look, but don't overpower you, giving the clothes more emphasis than the man. For example, a light person with blonde hair wearing a dark navy suit will wash out or fade into the background.

Following are lists of recommended shirt and tie combinations with navy and gray suits for all coloring. Added are recommended optional colors for suits that can be used for a less powerful presentation and in situations that do not require a "uniform" look. A universal color list is included on page 124 listing those colors that can be successfully worn by everyone since they are neither too dark or light, warm or cool, or muted or bright.

Remember that in industries such as fashion, advertising, and public relations, rules of dress are slightly more creative. Brown, beige, and often green suits are possible additions to your wardrobe. It is preferable that the browns be tweeds, tone-on-tone or textured for the most professional appearance. Beiges range from warm golden beige to a taupe or gray-beige color. You can select the beige or tan that is most complementary to your skintone and as described in the color charts.

YOUR COLOR I.Q.

You can wear all colors. Recognizing the best ones for your wardrobe is essential to complement your personal characteristics. Here is a basic primer on the terminology of color that you'll need to know to get the most our of Chapter Eight.

Bright vs. Muted

Brightness is a characteristic of color that describes how brilliant or dull a color is. Each color has bright or muted qualities. Muted colors have been softened by adding gray to lessen intensity.

Deep vs. Light

Depth is a characteristic of color that describes how light or dark a color is. Consider any color from its darkest shade to its lightest and all the ones in between.

Warm vs. Cool

The undertone of a color determines whether a color is warm or cool. Warm colors are yellow- or gold-based. Cool colors are more blue-based. It is easy to see when you compare two tones of the same color side-by-side. The one that looks more yellow is the warmer tone. The one that looks more blue is the cooler.

COLORS FOR MEN WITH WARM COLORING

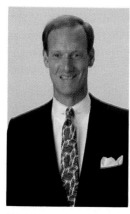

SHIRTS　　　NEUTRALS　　　ACCENTS & CASUALS

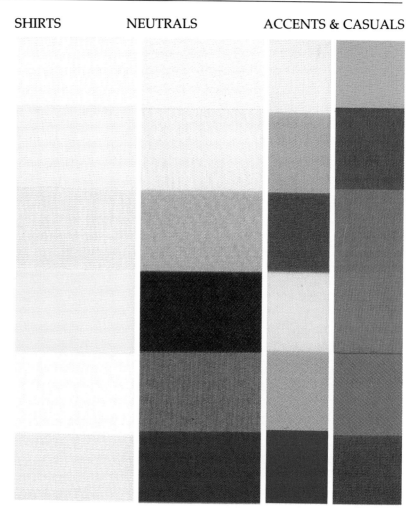

WARM   The "warm" person projects a total golden glow. There will be evidence of a true golden undertone in the hair, eyes, and skin tone. If you can describe your coloring as warm you will always be successful wearing warm-based colors of medium depth.

See in Chapter seven for the full description of skintones, hair, and eye colors typical of this color group. Physical characteristics, colors to avoid, and suggested shirt and tie combinations for men with Warm coloring are also listed in this chapter.

COLORS FOR SHIRTS (*left column*). Stripes in Accent & Casual colors can be used with white and other shirt colors (*listed top to bottom*):Icy pink, Icy blue, Icy violet, Icy aqua, Icy yellow, Apricot.

NEUTRALS   (*second column from left, top to bottom*):Ivory, Light warm beige, Camel, Medium golden brown, Gray, Marine navy.

ACCENTS & CASUAL (*right columns top to bottom*): Buff, Pumpkin, Terra cotta, Yellow-gold, Deep peach/apricot, Orange-red, Bright yellow-green, Teal, Turquoise, Emerald turquoise, Deep periwinkle blue, Purple.

SHIRTS NEUTRALS ACCENTS & CASUALS

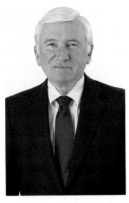

COOL The "cool" person often has a rose or pink complexion. It is often described as rosey. Cool coloring in general will be the mid-tone range, neither too dark nor light. Few young people are best described as cool. But often as people age, coloring lightens or softens. Many youthful "brights" or "deeps" become cool as their hair grays.

See Chapter Seven for the full description of skintones, hair, and eye colors typical of this color group. Physical characteristics, colors to avoid, and suggested shirt and tie combinations for men with cool coloring are also listed in this chapter.

COLORS FOR SHIRTS *(left column)*. These colors are standard shirt colors for solids and stripes. The "cool" person should avoid icy aqua and apricot. Stripes in Accent & Casual colors can be used with white and other shirt colors *(listed top to bottom)*:Icy pink, Icy blue, Icy violet, Icy aqua, Icy yellow, Apricot.

NEUTRALS *(second column from left, top to bottom)*:Soft white, Medium true gray, Charcoal blue-gray, Gray-beige (taupe), Cocoa, Navy,

ACCENTS & CASUAL *(right columns top to bottom)*: Light lemon yellow, Royal blue, Medium blue, Deep blue-green, Emerald green, Deep rose, Shocking pink, Deep hot pink, Burgundy, Blue-red, Raspberry, Royal purple.

SHIRTS   NEUTRALS   ACCENTS & CASUALS

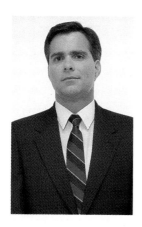

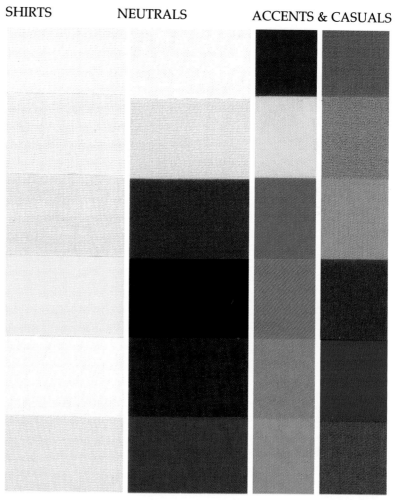

DEEP The "deep" person's color characteristic is the easiest to see. Do you have dark eyes and dark hair? If so, you are deep. There are warm and cool undertones in the deep person, and he can successfully wear deep colors that are neither too blue nor too gold.

See Chapter Seven for the full description of skintones, hair, and eye colors typical of this color group. Physical characteristics, colors to avoid, and suggested shirt and tie combinations for men with deep coloring are also listed in this chapter.

COLORS FOR SHIRTS *(left column)*. These colors are standard shirt colors for solids and stripes. Stripes in Accent & Casual colors can be used with white and other shirt colors *(listed top to bottom)*:Icy pink, Icy blue, Icy violet, Icy aqua, Icy yellow, Apricot.

NEUTRALS   *(second column from left, top to bottom)*:Oyster white, Gray-beige (taupe), Charcoal gray, Black, Dark chocolate brown, Navy.

ACCENTS & CASUAL *(right columns top to bottom):* Mahogany, Yellow gold, True blue, Deep periwinkle blue, Chinese blue, Hot turquoise, Teal, Salmon, True green, Pine green, True red, Purple.

SHIRTS   NEUTRALS   ACCENTS & CASUALS

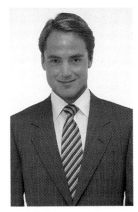

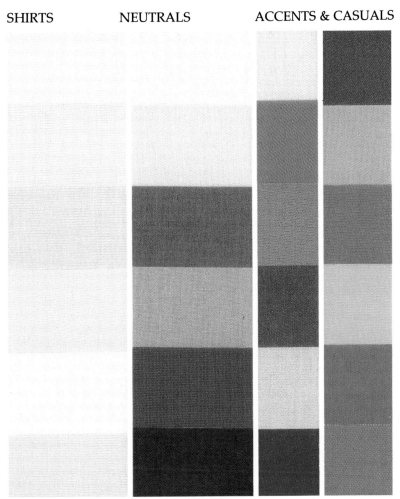

LIGHT The "light" person has light hair color—blonde—, golden or ash—medium to dark. Your hair may darken when not exposed to sunlight and then rapidly lighten as bleached by the sun. There will be little contrast between hair color and skin tone. Eyes will be blue, green, or appear to change from blue to green with the colors you are wearing.

See Chapter Seven for the full description of skintones, hair, and eye colors typical of this color group. Physical characteristics, colors to avoid, and suggested shirt and tie combinations for men with light coloring are also listed in this chapter.

COLORS FOR SHIRTS (*left column*). These colors are standard shirt colors for solids and stipes. Stripes in Accent & Casual colors can be used with white and other shirt colors (*listed top to bottom*):Icy pink, Icy blue, Icy violet, Icy aqua, Icy yellow, Apricot.

NEUTRALS (*second column from left, top to bottom*):Soft white, Light warm beige, Cocoa, Light warm gray, Charcoal blue-gray, Grayed navy.

ACCENTS & CASUAL (*right columns top to bottom*) Buff, Deep blue-green, Coral pink, Clear bright warm pink, Powder pink, Deep rose, Watermelon, Light warm aqua, Emerald turquoise, Sky blue, Periwinkle, Medium blue.

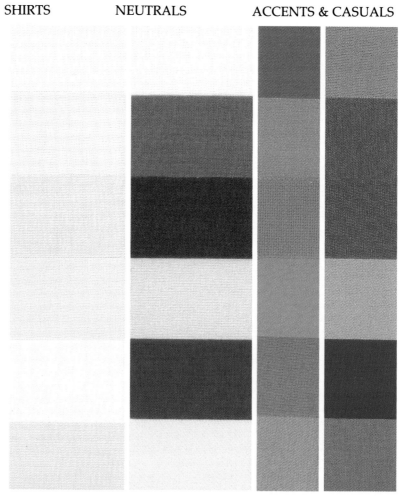

SHIRTS NEUTRALS ACCENTS & CASUALS

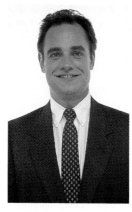

BRIGHT The "bright" person has a crisp look derived from a strong contrast between skin and hair color and the jewel-like clarity of the eye color. Eyes will be blue, green, Turquoise, but are *not* brown.

See Chapter Seven for the full description of skintones, hair, and eye colors typical of this color group. Physical characteristics, colors to avoid, and suggested shirt and tie combinations for men with bright coloring are also listed in this chapter.

COLORS FOR SHIRTS *(left column)*. These colors are standard shirt colors for solids and stripes. Stripes in Accent & Casual colors can be used with white and other shirt colors *(listed top to bottom):*Icy pink, Icy blue, Icy violet, Icy aqua, Icy yellow, Apricot.

NEUTRALS *(second column from left, top to bottom):*Soft white, Medium true gray, Charcoal gray, Gray-beige (taupe), Navy, Lemon Yellow.

ACCENTS & CASUAL *(right columns top to bottom):* True blue, Dark periwinkle blue, Chinese blue, Hot turquoise, True green, Coral pink, Clear bright pink, Deep hot pink, Shocking pink, True red, Medium violet.

COLORS FOR MEN WITH MUTED COLORING

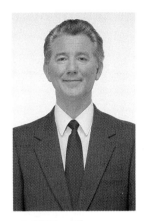

SHIRTS   NEUTRALS   ACCENTS & CASUALS

MUTED The "muted" person is neither light nor dark, but has coloring that is medium in depth. Hair color will be light, ash blonde, ash brown or medium blonde. With light hair, eyes will be brown, hazel or teal (blue-green). The main difference between the muted and light will be the eye color that projects warmth and richness to the overall presentation.

See Chapter Seven for the full description of skintones, hair, and eye colors typical of this color group. Physical characteristics, colors to avoid, and suggested shirt and tie combinations for men with muted coloring are also listed in this chapter.

COLORS FOR SHIRTS *(left column)*. These colors are standard shirt colors for solids and stripes. Stripes in Accent & Casual colors can be used with white and other shirt colors *(listed top to bottom)*:Icy pink, Icy blue, Icy violet, Icy aqua, Icy yellow, Apricot.

NEUTRALS *(second column from left, top to bottom)*:Soft white, Rose beige, Cocoa, Coffee brown, Marine navy, Charcoal blue-gray.

ACCENTS & CASUAL *(right columns top to bottom)*: Mahogany, Light lemon yellow, Periwinkle, Deep blue-green, Grayed green, Olive green, Teal, Turquoise, Deep rose, Salmon, Watermelon, Purple.

TIES AND SHIRTS: WHAT GOES WITH WHAT?

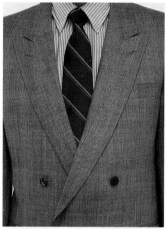

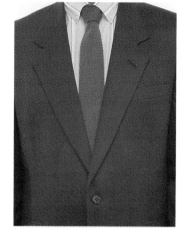

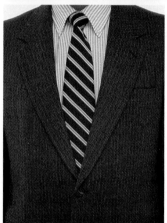

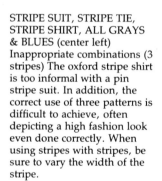

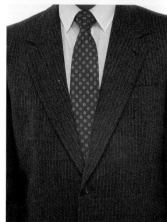

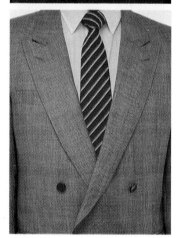

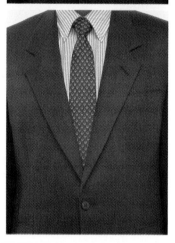

DARK GRAY SINGLE BREASTED, GREEN TIE (top right) This knit tie and casual striped shirt should be worn with a sport coat or blazer. They are too casual for the suit.

LIGHT GRAY DOUBLE BREASTED, TEAL STRIPE TIE (top left) The oxford stripe is too casual for the double-breasted sharp-straight silhouette. The three patterns are not compatible. A widely spaced fine stripe shirt in broadcloth would work well for a fashionable look.

DARK GRAY PIN STRIPE SINGLE, RED DOT TIE (center right) A correct use of the oxford shirt with a foulard tie. (1 solid, 2 patterns)

STRIPE SUIT, STRIPE TIE, STRIPE SHIRT, ALL GRAYS & BLUES (center left) Inappropriate combinations (3 stripes) The oxford stripe shirt is too informal with a pin stripe suit. In addition, the correct use of three patterns is difficult to achieve, often depicting a high fashion look even done correctly. When using stripes with stripes, be sure to vary the width of the stripe.

STRIPE SUIT, STRIPE SHIRT, ALL GRAYS & BLUES, RED DOT TIE (bottom right) (1 solid, 2 patterns) A correct combination of a pin stripe suit and geometric design on tie.

LIGHT GRAY DOUBLE BREASTED SUIT, RED STRIPE TIE (bottom left) (1 solid, 2 patterns) This is a correct look: solid with stripe with glenn plaid.

✓ COLOR CHECKLIST

Color is one of our most important characteristics and choosing the right ones can make all the difference. Improvising without guidelines may be fun but you can wind up looking like a painter's palette. To focus your style and blend your colors to your special needs, review the following checklist:

☐ Colors, like line, scale, and fit must complement you physically, express your personality, be appropriate for the occasion, and must be current.

☐ Colors affect your complexion — wrinkles seem to disappear, circles under the eyes are less noticeable, five o'clock shadows disappear, and eye color is brightened. Understanding your best colors will ensure a healthy, young looking, credible look.

☐ Color projects different signals. Deep colors project authority and power. Medium and light colors are more friendly and informal. Although colors themselves send out messages, they are being worn by *you*. Therefore, it is necessary to understand just how dark and light your colors can be to create the mood you want without overpowering you or making you look insignificant.

☐ Navy and gray are the classic suit colors. White and blue shirts are the most acceptable. They project a solid, conservative look.

☐ Other colors like tan, beige, brown, and green may be worn with care depending upon your coloring and the occasion. Bright colors and new color combinations are fine in small amounts or for more casual and dressed up times.

☐ Beige and tan are the preferred colors for raincoats.

☐ All color can be described by three characteristics: an undertone, warm or cool; a depth, dark or light; or intensity, bright or muted. By understanding colors and their characteristics it is possible to identify those that work with your coloring.

☐ Our skintone, hair, and eye color can also be described by the same three color characteristics: undertone, depth, and intensity. Each of us projects one characteristic more strongly than another so we can identify our coloring as warm, cool, deep, light, bright or muted and select the corresponding colors to create balance and harmony.

☐ You can wear all colors but it is important to combine them with other colors, as in shirts and tie combinations. Just be sure the combinations are right for you.

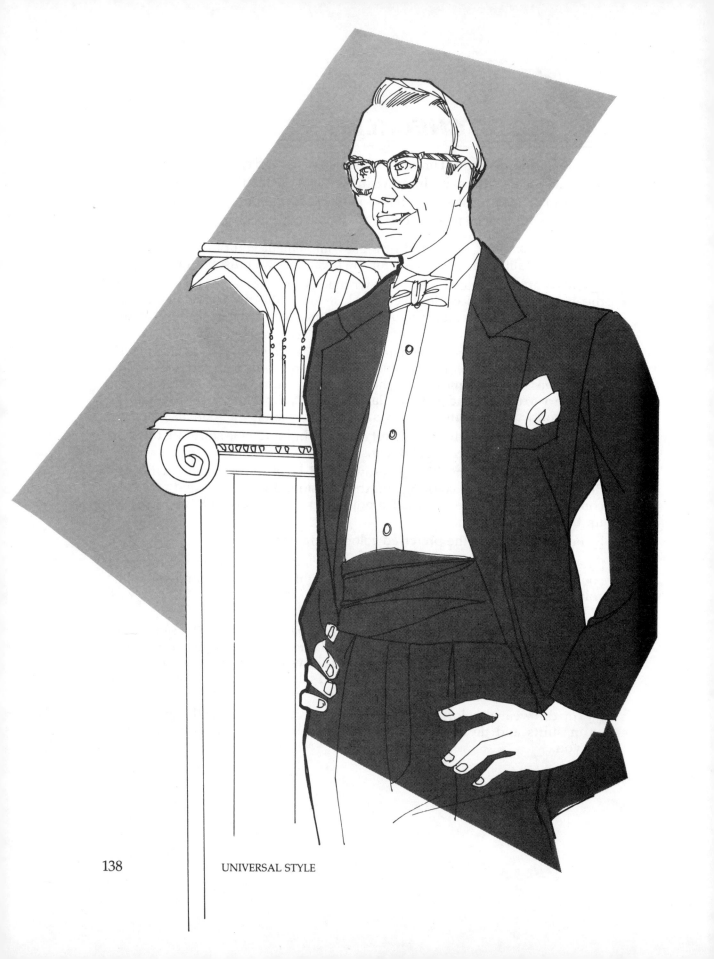

UNIVERSAL STYLE

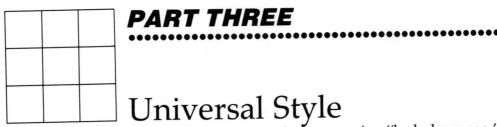

PART THREE

Universal Style

In this section we're going to examine "body language," the silent voice that often says more about you than words. How you fill the space around you is important to your overall style. Now you'll find out what you're doing right and — heaven forbid! — wrong.

There is also a complete primer of business etiquette and protocol. Though it's controversial and still very much a changing scene, we'll pinpoint the essentials of etiquette U.S.A., including dining and travel tips and what the new working woman expects from her "New Age" male colleagues.

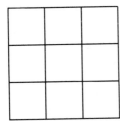

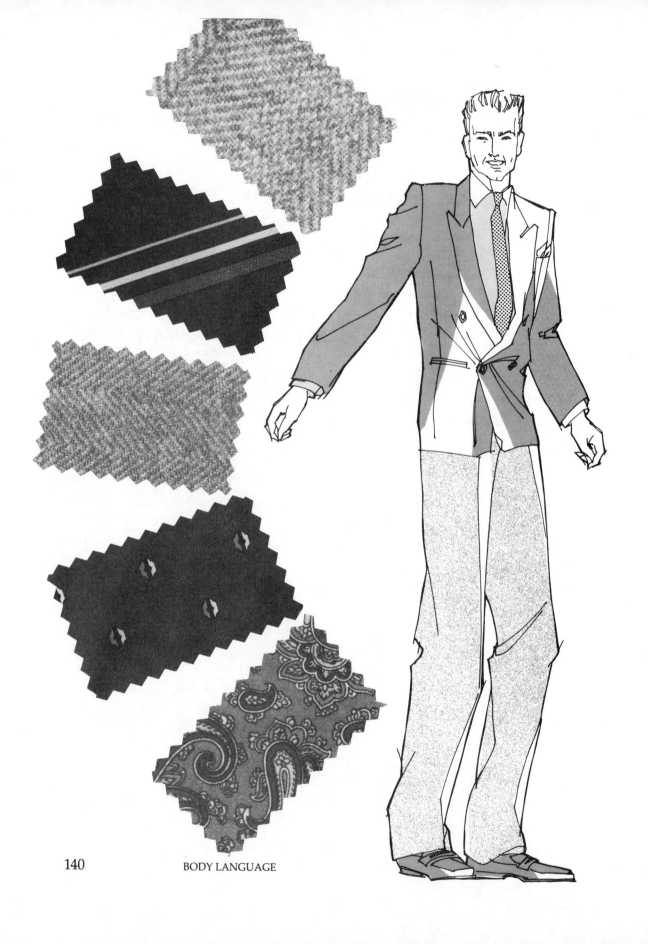

140   BODY LANGUAGE

CHAPTER EIGHT

BODY LANGUAGE

Filling The Space Around You

In the beginning of this book we focused mostly on how to dress, on your immediate image. This chapter is more personal. It looks at who you are and how you occupy the space around you.

It's called body language. The *American Heritage Dictionary* defines this as, "The bodily gestures, postures, and facial expressions by which an individual communicates non-verbally with others." Thirty years ago, body language wasn't in most dictionaries. Today it's an industry.

If progress is what we've made, body language has become a part of it. Space communication dishes and mass media have made us aware of looks on a grand scale. When we watch the President of the United States during a televised press conference we're aware of each subtle nuance. Did he look uncomfortable in front of the microphone? Did he tremble just a bit? Or was he projecting confidence through his body language? We pay a lot less attention to what he actually has to say. Could it be that what we see is more important to us than what someone may be trying to say?

We'll leave the verbal projection up to you. You're pretty expert at it, since no one knows your world better than you do. Our concentration will be on the non-verbal, the body language that sometimes says more about you than your most carefully chosen words.

Body Language in Business

It's easy to lose sight of body language in the workplace. That's because we tend to believe that our assigned duties and built-in office protocol act as a buffer between ourselves and our colleagues. Yet body language is critical to the way we conduct business. It's a vital element of total presentation and style and it may have profound impact on the success or failure of any given situation.

The importance of body language is most obvious in the charged atmosphere of meeting someone for the first time. You enter someone's office feeling good about your outward appearance — your clothes and grooming — but within 30 seconds or less, impressions start to change. Perhaps you slouch in the chair, cross and uncross your legs, express a lack of ease with your hands, or lean on the other person's desk. These signals can overpower even the most meticulous outward appearance.

Let's examine some of the more important elements of body language:

Posture: When you slouch, either standing or seated, you generate at least five negative signals: *lack of confidence, indifference, low self-esteem, tiredness, or just plain sloppiness.* It isn't necessary to maintain a military bearing, but you do want to project alertness and attention to what's going on around you. Also, good posture minimizes distracting gestures and lets you concentrate more fully on the business at hand.

Eye contact: Perhaps more important than posture is good eye contact. Nothing is more unnerving than someone who refuses to look you in the eye. Maintaining good eye contact (not a penetrating stare!) projects *integrity, honesty, self-confidence, and genuine interest in the other person.* Wandering eyes indicate nervousness, indifference, or boredom. Good contact demands 95 percent of your time; anything less may be a clear signal that you're in a losing position.

Handshakes: The first physical movement in most business settings is a handshake. In meeting another man, a firm hand- shake (no bone-crushers!) and good eye contact get things off to a positive start. When shaking hands with a woman, tone down the firmness, but not to the extent of presenting her with a "dead fish." If you wear heavy rings on your right hand make certain they don't dig into the hand you're holding. Two other small points: when someone enters your office, rise and extend your hand in greeting. A proper greeting projects *confidence, control, and honesty.*

Unacceptable handshakes: The two-handed clasp, popularized by the late President Lyndon B. Johnson (and used frequently by politicians), is inappropriate and inconsistent in a business atmosphere. It is especially condescending in male/female introductions. Sweaty palms are also a turn-off. For a confident, take-charge greeting, be the first to extend your hand.

Too close for comfort: Respect space. Don't "cozy-up" to someone with whom you're engaged in a one-on-one conversation. This is especially critical in male/female situations where personal sensitivities can run high. One's "personal zone" of inviolate space is generally 18 inches to three feet around them. This is safe for cocktail parties and other social or casual events. Three to five feet is the correct business distance, but six feet is considered "distant" or "aloof." These spacing guidelines apply to standing greetings, walking up to someone's desk, or coming up behind someone.

When it comes to looking over documents, papers, or other materials, it's best to make duplicate copies to avoid invasion of your colleague's "personal zone." The comfort that results, along with the signal of being prepared, adds positive points to your total presentation.

Touching: Outside of visiting a good pal or the standard business handshake, the rule is: *No touching!* It's an invasion of space. It's also confusing. What's the purpose of touching in a business situation? Just how friendly are you anyway? *And never touch a female business associate!* It's guaranteed to generate all the wrong impressions.

The avoidance of touching also extends to inanimate objects, such as decorations (especially paintings), or small show pieces on someone's desk. Unless requested to "just feel the weight of this desk set," practice a strict hands-off policy.

Skillful listening: Have you ever noticed that the best conversationalists are also the best listeners? Listening is a conscious art; it takes no small amount of discipline, particularly when dealing with less than articulate people. Always look at the other person and notice the inflections of voice. Listen for content and allow full expression of ideas before making a reply. If you don't understand something, ask questions. When you don't agree with a point-of-view, stay cool; let the person finish, then try to summarize what they've said, just to make sure you've received an accurate message. Ignore distractions and/or confusing, irrelevant twists of conversation. Don't tune them out entirely — there may be a good idea hidden in the maze — but focus on the central issues.

Other points of skillful listening involve appropriate feedback. Let the speaker know you get the message. If a person is slow or halting in speech, *do not* give in to the temptation of completing their sentences for them. It is a clear sign of impatience and rudeness. Almost as bad is looking at your watch during a conversation or fidgeting in your seat. And, unless invited to do so, don't smoke.

Reading Body Language

Every day we're in contact with people, casually or professionally. We listen to what they have to say, but we're also in the position of having to put their words together with non-verbal clues to get the full message.

Below is a short course on reading the meaning behind the most commonly used body language.

Receiving Positive Signals

- [ ] Smiles, laughs, in a natural, unforced way.
- [ ] **Makes reference to, or shows you, objects of personal interest,** such as pictures of family, awards, letters from colleagues.
- [ ] **When** you sit across the desk, the other party clears away papers and other **objects that come between you.**
- [ ] Maintains eye contact.
- [ ] When speaking to you, the other person keeps hands away from face.
- [ ] Has straight posture. The person leans toward you when speaking.
- [ ] Makes easy, loose gestures; is relaxed while seated or standing.
- [ ] Allows meeting to run slightly overtime.
- [ ] **Listens, then makes quick notes on the important points you wish to get across.**
- [ ] Stands and walks you to the door when the meeting is over.

Receiving Negative Signals

- [ ] Little or no eye contact.
- [ ] Squinting, furrows appear on the brow.
- [ ] Has cool, too-quick handshake.
- [ ] Places hands anywhere on face.
- [ ] Looks at the floor, walls, or desktop.
- [ ] **Clenches hands, drums on desktop; makes nervous or impatient movement of hands.**
- [ ] Has tight-set mouth; little or no smile.
- [ ] Rigid posture, with feet flat on the floor.
- [ ] Keeps checking wrist watch.
- [ ] Allows incoming calls to continually break the flow of conversation.
- [ ] Acts distracted, vague, clearly preoccupied.
- [ ] Silently conveys a sense of aloofness.

THE GROOMED LOOK OF SUCCESS

Grooming

This is not an example of a corporate executive on his way to the top (right). The signals being sent out are more of an artist or surfer, etc. This may be fine for the day off but he should be able to make the transition from work to play to formal.

(Below right) Appropriate beard, moustache, and hair style if acceptable in your industry or company.

(Below left) This clean shaven look shows the entire face and is considered the most professional.

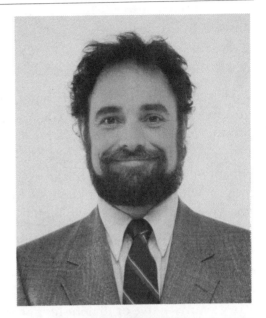

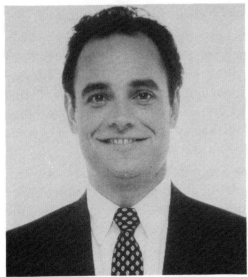

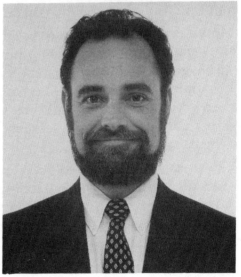

Notes on beards and mustache - many studies have been done confirming that a clean shaven face projects more credibility, honesty and is therefore preferable in a corporate setting. Some companies allow for well-trimmed and maintained beards.

Clearly, body language presents a challenge. It is infinitely diverse and varies with people, settings, cultures, situations; it's a life-long study. The more aware you become, the more you learn to read the signals and project those that help you make it to the top. Best of all, it's fun. And, as a business skill, it's downright invaluable.

Making It Into the Front Office

This section deals with body language *and* verbal signals. The setting is the reception area of Mega-Corp. Your mission is to sell yourself or your company's product to Mister Big, the vice-president in charge of just about everything.

By now, of course, you realize that the impression you make at Mega-Corp began when you phoned for an appointment. You made all the right verbal moves, which is what got you here in the first place. And now that you're in, you've got to keep the image high.

Time spent in the reception area is important. When you enter, introduce yourself pleasantly to the receptionist. Give your name, title, affiliation, and the name of the person you're there to see, along with the time of the appointment. Your business card is an added bonus. Present it upon arrival. Arrive early — five or 10 minutes ahead — and acknowledge that you're a few minutes ahead of time. Sure, you can wait; you've got a bit of reading to do.

If you're wearing an overcoat, ask the receptionist where to stow it. You want your hands free for the upcoming introductions. In most cases, the receptionist will hang up your coat. This may seem terribly obvious and not worth worrying about, but this little gesture is both functional and subtle. It sends a signal that you're accustomed to being in places where your coat (and hat, if you wear one) has been taken care of. In a very quiet way, it says you've been around in some of the better places.

View your time in the reception area as a mini-rehearsal for your visit with Mister Big. Set your mood and tone. Scrub out any indications of boredom or anxiety; start pumping up the old enthusiasm and self-confidence. Chat to the receptionist about nothing much in general. Be congenial and relaxed; make certain all your systems are "go."

You may be a bit on edge, but don't smoke. There's too much controversy about lighting up, and controversy is exactly what you don't need. The receptionist may be puffing away. That's okay, *but not for you*. If the receptionist offers you a soft drink or coffee, politely decline. Thanks but no thanks. You don't want a cup or glass in your hand when Mister Big — or Mister Big's assistant — arrives to usher you into the inner sanctum.

STANDING UP FOR YOURSELF

Right and Wrong Posture

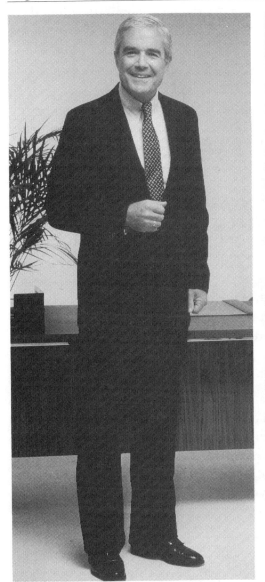 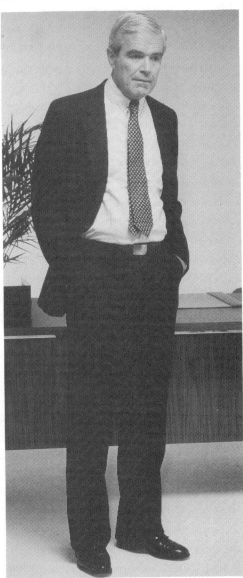

As well-dressed as Leo is (right), his slumped posture and stance send out a message. He may be thinking and comfortable. However when getting ready for an introduction, he looks too relaxed and perhaps bored.

(Left) In preparation for an introduction, meeting, or presentation, his buttoned suit, straight posture, and stance say confidence, control, and power.

Once your meeting begins, it's fine to accept coffee or whatever else may be offered. Fine, that is, if the others are going to join you. If Mister Big is also taking up time with a cup of coffee, so be it. But don't go solo. You want to make every second count, and it's easy to let a lot of time slip by while deciding if you want milk, cream, "Creamora," sugar, or "Nutrasweet." Taking it black is better, but time is still slipping away.

Introductions are always advisable in a business setting. Unless you're very familiar with the person you're meeting, it's a good idea to introduce yourself and spell out your position. I never assume that someone will remember my name. I may be overly sensitive on this point, but personally I have difficulty remembering names. Faces and events are different, I rarely forget them. But I'm not fully at ease until I know the names of all the players and make sure they know who I am.

It's certainly the place of Mister Big to be prepared, stand, extend his hand in greeting, and welcome you by name. If not, it's up to you. If you've come with your colleagues, introduce the "lesser" to the "mightier." Between men and women of equal age and status, protocol allows whatever is most comfortable. However, I feel it's appropriate to follow the rules of corporate etiquette and introduce by rank regardless of sex. Once the introductions are out of the way, mention the approximate length of your visit: "I believe we can present our product (or service) to you in about 10 minutes . . . " Having said that, the scene is completely set.

You're now going to do a lot of talking — selling, really — and body quirks shouldn't get in the way.

Sit with correct posture, relaxed and comfortable, but with a kind of forward lean toward the business you're doing. If possible, avoid low, soft-cushioned sofas or chairs, especially if Mister Big is propped confidently behind the desk in a high straight-back chair. You want to feel "on a level" — eye-to eye — so you can play on the same turf. Ideally, you want to be directly across the desk so that eye contact can be maintained.

Some people feel this "on a level" approach isn't terribly critical. After all, they say, they've gotten this far and no silly chair or seating arrangement is going to keep them from closing the deal. Well, maybe not. But why risk it, short of there being no other alternative? The next time you watch a television talk show, notice how the host is invariably seated in a higher position than the guests. The reason is that the host, the star, is projecting status to the viewing audience. If it didn't work, it wouldn't be practiced by so many talk show hosts, who, it must be said, are playing for ratings and millions of dollars.

Back to Mister Big.

THE LOOK OF CONFIDENCE

Right and Wrong Eye Contact

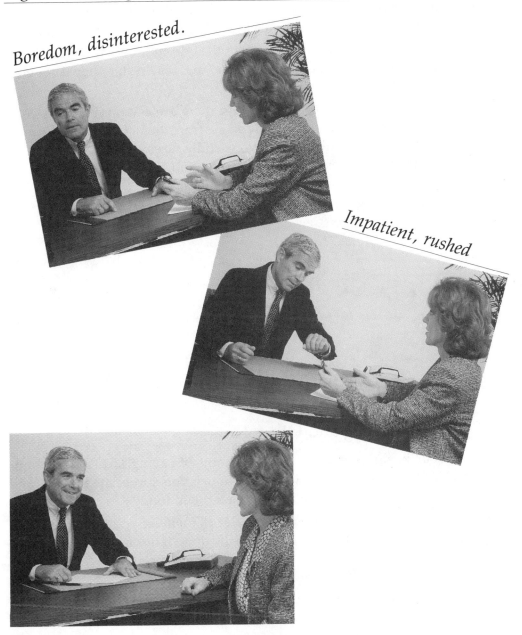

Boredom, disinterested.

Impatient, rushed

Looking at your watch during a conversation is rude. Hold all calls unless it is an emergency.

Correct eye contact is pleasant, confident, and respectful.

Use the dynamics of business "power seating" to your advantage. "Power seating" is corporate jargon for strategic placement in a room. For example, at a rectangular conference table with the head position representing the "authority figure," persons seated in positions (chairs) three, five, and seven are in the best position to achieve eye contact with the leader.

Because of this dynamic, those seated in the odd-numbered chairs will gain the most attention from the "authority figure" and, as a result, they'll be able to dominate the scene.

If you're in a meeting with a group and there are certain members you'd rather avoid, don't seat yourself directly across from them. Choose a seat on the same side of the table, with one or two friendly faces between you. It's just enough of a barrier to avoid possible confrontation.

Sample Seating Arrangements

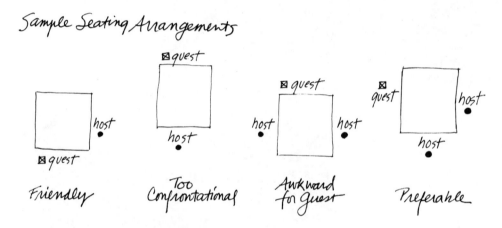

Friendly | Too Confrontational | Awkward for Guest | Preferable

So Long, Mister Big and Other Exits

When your business is done, make a point of saying so. Pack up your briefcase and let Mister Big know just how much you appreciate his time and attention. If assistants are in the room, thank them, too.

If you've made a good impression, Mister Big will let you know when he *stands* to shake your hand and walks you to the door. If he does neither of these things, his body language is sending troublesome signals.

Say goodbye to the assistants. Smile. Tell them how much you enjoyed meeting them, that you hope to see them again in the near future. While you're at it, check their body language for small, telling signals.

You may feel perfectly at home in Mister Big's office; perhaps there are indications that you should stick around a little longer to chat idly. *Don't even think about it!* Leave them wanting more.

EXTEND YOUR HAND

Right and Wrong Handshakes

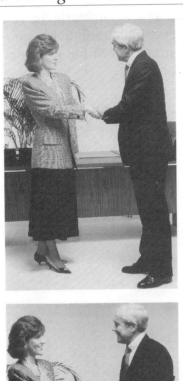
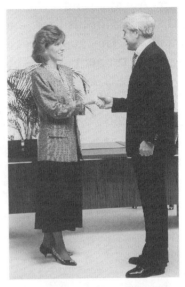
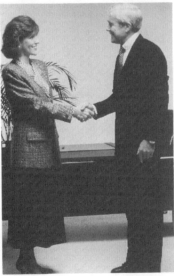
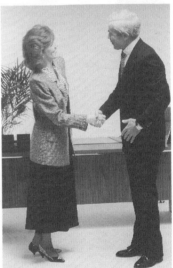

The timid, limp handshake (top right) is not acceptable for men or women. It says insecurity and lack of confidence.

The double-handshake (top left) is condescending and should not be used under any circumstances.

The bone crusher (bottom right) does not impress men or women regardless of your weight-lifting ability. Save that for the health club.

The correct handshake (bottom left) is firm, direct, and complementary.

Don't ignore the receptionist on the way out — and don't forget your coat. Pass out the thanks and the smiles. You want only good impressions to flow in your wake.

Follow up: Always send a follow-up letter summarizing your meeting, thanking Mister Big for his time, and specifically outlining your next step or your expectations. This guarantees a written record for you from a business standpoint and is proper business etiquette.

HOW CLOSE FOR COMFORT

Right and Wrong Territory

Once introductions are made, be careful of invading personal territory. This is too close and is better saved for intimate times.

Pointing fingers. This is often interpreted as dictatorial.

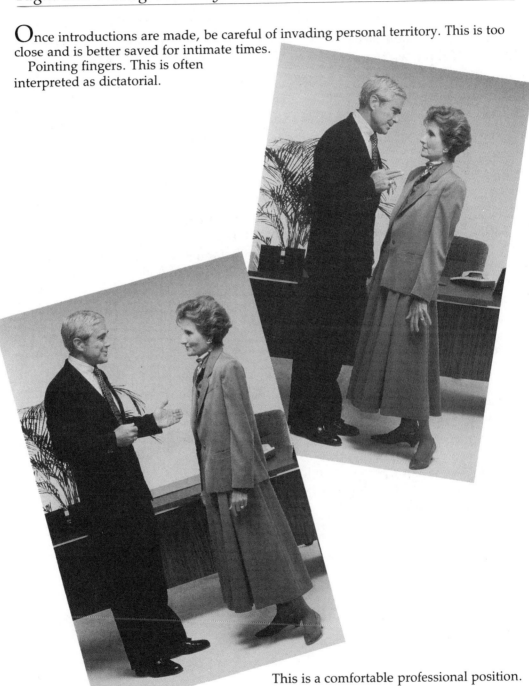

This is a comfortable professional position.

✔ BODY LANGUAGE CHECKLIST

Body language — it's universal! Everyone speaks it fluently.

Speaking is one thing, but understanding body language is a silent social science. People with any degree of awareness *work at learning it* because of its impact on our style, our own silent language that tells more about us than words.

The checklist is a primer for this science. By no means is it encyclopedic — it's a start, a road map to help you understand others and yourself, too.

☐ Body language is a non-verbal projection of personality and mood. Depending on signals sent, its impact may be positive or negative.

☐ The language creates "space" around its user. This space extends up to three feet around a person. Violating that space with unnecessary intrusions, no matter how well-meaning, sends bad signals about you.

☐ Touching in a business setting is generally limited to handshakes. Make it a firm handshake if you're meeting or greeting another male. Tone it down for women. Keep those palms dry!

☐ Retain good posture when seated, but maintain a relatively "easy" feeling about yourself. Remember, the day you were discharged from the service, your need for "military bearing" disappeared. The silent message is that you practice Good Manners-101.

☐ Eye contact is critical. It says you listen well and can hold attention when it's your turn to speak. Loss of contact during an interview is bad news. Don't stare down the person across the desk, but maintain eye contact 95 percent of the time.

☐ No matter how great you look, it's imperative to reinforce that look with the right body language. Together, personal appearance and body language are the essence of your personal style.

☐ Do you wear heavy rings? If so, remove them during work or be aware that one of your ordinary handshakes may be hazardous to someone else's health. Maybe your own.

☐ Unless expressly invited to do so, *don't smoke in meetings, other people's offices, or reception areas.* That habit carries negative signals.

☐ If you're a congressman from Washington you can be forgiven of one of those "LBJ two-fisted handshakes." Otherwise, the two-handed clasp is out of bounds in business. It's also offensive to many women.

☐ Before meeting a potential client or employer, practice the body language of alert relaxation. You can rehearse in the reception area by setting a mood with the receptionist. Don't be intrusive or distracting. A little thoughtful conversation is enough to set the mood.

☐ If you know a business associate well, an exchange of names isn't needed. But when meeting with someone new, make sure you introduce yourself and give your company affiliation.

☐ There are "power seats" around any rectangular conference table. The head of the table is the "authority figure" who makes the action happen. To be in a position to best gain the authority figure's attention, sit in seats three, five, and seven. These strategically located positions make it easy to maintain eye contact with the person at the head of the table.

☐ To avoid confrontations in a similar setting, it's a good idea to sit on the same side of the table as the person you hope to avoid. Put a couple of neutrals between you, if possible. Under such conditions, the lack of eye contact will keep a lid on things.

☐ Don't take body language for granted. It speaks even when we're unaware of it. Work to make the voice a positive one!

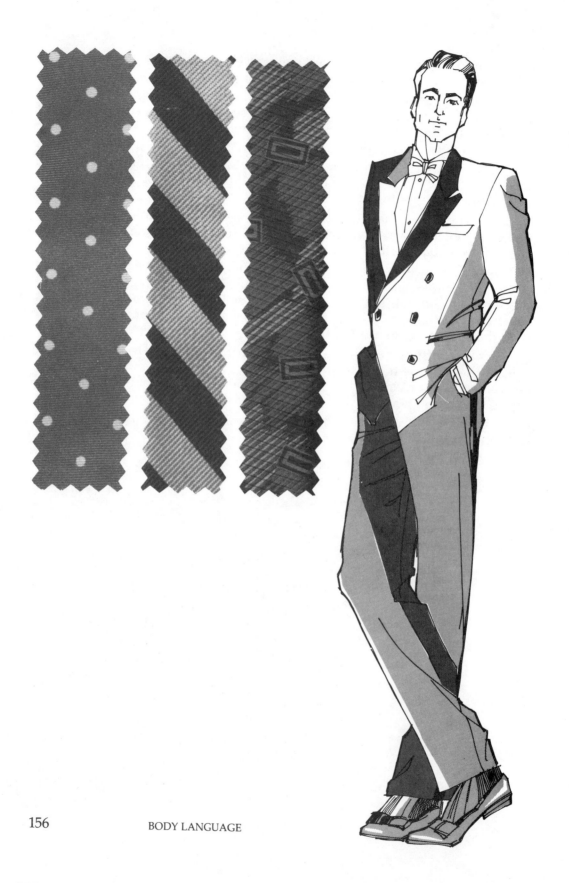

BODY LANGUAGE

CHAPTER NINE

LIVE
WIRE

Women And "New Age" Manners

Lisa S., quit her $3.75-an-hour job as a receptionist to manhandle a jackhammer at a construction site. When her boss, known as "Mack the Knife" because of his quick-tempered firing techniques, asked Lisa what she was doing on "man's turf," she told him: "I'm making four times the money I made on my last job, that's what!"

Unamused, "Mack the Knife" replied: "You'll get the money, baby, if you move a ton of concrete a day."

Lisa moved her daily ton of concrete all right, and when the boss handed her a check at the end of the first week, he apologized for having doubted her abilities. "You're okay," he said. "Like a skinny guy."

"Sure," Lisa said. "No hard feelings."

When another worker touched her, she didn't complain to "Mack the Knife." She didn't file a complaint with an attorney or the Equal Employment Opportunities Commission. She simply smacked him hard enough to send his hardhat flying. "No hard feelings," she told him.

Lisa isn't exactly a total embodiment of today's "New Wave" woman, but she's close. Consider a more genteel example, Sarah S., a 31-year-old marketing expert:

Not long ago Sarah invited a prospective client, Jason V., to lunch in hopes of landing a contract for her services. She was confident she could find new ways to market Jason's software packages.

It was a productive meeting — productive, that is, until the bill arrived. Jason launched into a well-meaning but bellicose "allow me" routine. He bullied the waiter into handing him the tab, and, with the waiter looking on, he joked, "Men pay for the ladies, right?"

Wrong! Sarah had done the inviting in the first place. Before Jason arrived she'd told the waiter to take an impression of her credit card, which she'd sign when the bill was tallied. Jason's behavior caused no small amount of embarrassment (Sarah was a regular at the restaurant). In addition, Jason left the distinct — and fatal — impression that he was an incurable "male chauvinist."

In the end, Sarah passed up the deal because she felt his behavior at the restaurant was a precursor of things to come. She simply couldn't chance launching herself on what appeared to be a collision course. As for Jason, he was left with the hollow feeling of having committed a serious *faux pas*, though he never did figure out what he'd done wrong.

Lisa and Sarah are important to you because they represent nearly 60 percent of the workforce, the cadre of women age 21 to 35 who are striving to take charge of middle and upper management by the turn of the century. They're here to stay. We hope this discussion will help you survive in style with your competitive "sisters."

A New Wave Profile

Unlike the previous generation, the New Wavers tend to be fiercely independent, risk takers, aggressive, tough; traits not associated with the social or romantic side of women.

There are other salient attributes. The New Wavers are typically well-educated and, on average, score higher in IQ tests than their male counterparts. They're also athletic and competitive, smart where a previous generation might have been "cunning" (a word many New Wave women detest as sexist). They are politically aware and active on social issues. They do not believe that power, war, and politics are strictly male domains.

These women happen to be a majority of the population in America and, on the downside, they face a critical shortage of eligible young men. As a result, they're career-oriented, and they find no insurmountable problems when it comes to being single parents. The more traditional roles of wife and mother have become secondary for many; these aren't the crowning attainments they once were. If they can handle jackhammers and orbit in space, women feel they're fit to duke it out in the male jungle of competition and reward.

Even though males are harder to find, the New Wavers eschew much of traditional "femininity." When today's women do marry and bear children, their ambitions often remain intact. They may alter direction, but not their drive. And when it comes to money, it matters little or not at all that they may earn more of it than their husbands. Like Lisa, the attitude is, "No hard feelings."

What's A Man To Do?

Today's young men are every bit as ambitious as females, but when it comes to "handling" women — or, more precisely, when they must interact on a professional level — they are on skiddish ground. They're confused, and with good reason. A whole new ethic is at work, and it has little to do with old-fashioned values and courtesy, the very values most men are raised with. For better or worse, the time-honored role model of Sir Walter Raleigh, who spread his silk jacket across a puddle to allow a fair lady to pass spotlessly on her way, has suffered a fatal blow. These days Sir Walter is as archaic as a courtly bow or polite tip of the old fedora.

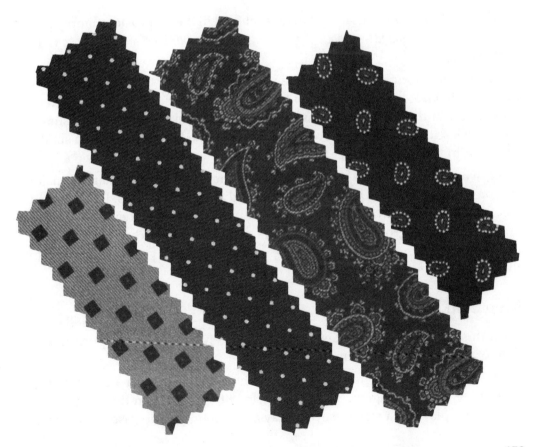

One of the most important things to remember is that in the midst of all this seeming chaos there's a distinct upside advantage for men. Today's protocol has liberated them from the gloomy (and often unfair) responsibility of always having to think, "ladies first." If the *Titanic* sank today, our New Wave women would (ideally) have no part of that noble admonition of the sea: "Women and children first." Once you understand that the women of the 1980's are charged with pulling their own weight over a variety of formerly male terrains, the world of work becomes a brighter, more amenable place to live.

What Do Women Want?

It's a tough question, but an answer may be at hand. At the turn of the century, Sigmund Freud, father of modern psychoanalysis, posed the question in print, with more than a little frustration. Most of his patients were well-to-do women with too much time on their hands. No matter how insightful or therapeutic he may have been in his practice, he found it next to impossible to quell the discontent. His immortal cry, "What does a woman want?" grew out of this experience.

Today the answer seems more tangible, at least in the workplace. Simply put, *women want — demand! — both the rewards and the burdens of equality, and no hard feelings.*

The demand seems only reasonable when you consider that women do two-thirds of all office work, represent a majority of the workforce and the general population, and yet hold down fewer than a third of all management positions and own less than one percent of the property in the U.S. If men had a similar situation in life, they'd gripe, too.

No wonder women are getting tougher. They are asked to handle major responsibilities, but find themselves devalued as human beings. Despite their recent social gains, women have the dubious distinction of being the fastest growing poverty group in America. The war of the sexes has gone slightly nuclear. If modern women appear to be warriors, men may take consolation in the fact that their assessment is right on the money.

Men Strike Back

Confused and/or infuriated by what they perceive to be female "pushiness," men of all ages have gone on the offensive.

Consider what happened to Ruth W., who was recently on a business trip with three male colleagues. The men carried little more than their briefcases. Ruth, who planned a stay of several days, was toting a briefcase, handbag, carry on luggage, and a heavy suitcase. At no time did her traveling companions offer a helping hand. Were there any hard feelings here? You bet, she said. "These men were in effect saying to me, 'You're one of us. You have a similar job description and you make the same money. So carry the bags yourself!'" "It was silly. If the tables were turned, I would have helped them — and I know they would have helped each other."

Apparently this was a case of sexism, resentment, and plain rudeness. Yet, in all fairness, men sometimes have good reason to act this way.

Paul Z., a Chicago-based public relations specialist, remembers a time when he would routinely give up his seat on the bus to a lady. Not any longer.

"If you're traditional, like me," Paul explains, "women think you're trying to put the move on them or that you've lost your mind."

He is by no means alone. We know of cases in which men have offered to light a lady's cigarette only to have the lighter batted out of their hands. Coat-holding has evoked similar reactions. The traditional male gesture of holding open doors is sometimes viewed by women as just another chauvinist insult. One client was raked by verbal fire when he tried to play doorman on a crowded Manhattan street. "Never again," he swore. "Let 'em wait."

The offenses and counter-offenses are so frequent that Abigail Van Buren, who writes the "Dear Abby" column, almost gives up: "If a person is kind or generous, it's an event."

Radio psychologist Toni Grant believes that the need for women to succeed in an economy that requires constant striving has had noticeable effects on male/female interaction. Women aren't entirely to blame for the breakdown in courtesy, she says, but the need to compete has raised a red flag.

"Women have traditionally created a climate for courtesy," she explains. "If you have a generation of hard-driving women, you don't have anyone holding the torch for social graces."

Judith Martin, known to her readers as "Miss Manners," believes we're "half a step above rock bottom" when it comes to politeness. There is, however, a glimmering of light. "If nothing else has happened, at least the problem has been identified."

Business Versus Social Protocol

Prior to the 1960's, there wasn't much difference between protocol in or outside the business environment, at least not where women were concerned. Men were either unabashedly rude or polite to women, in the office or outside of it. They believed in the words of an old song that "Men are men and women are women…in high silk hose and peek-a-boo clothes…" Clearly this was an attitude just begging to be shattered, which is exactly what happened in the wake of "Flower Power" and modern feminism.

Men were faced with a new ethic. Outside the office women demanded respect without the frills. Inside the business world they demanded, and received in law, equal status with men. The traditional use of "wiles" was scorned by the feminists. Women were competent or incompetent. Period. No tricks! Nowhere was this more evident than in the workplace. Competition, on equal grounds, was the ideal. Over time, relations between the sexes were reconstituted along more balanced lines. Outside of work men and women settled for a more gentle (and civil) coexistence, but on the job strict business protocol prevailed. It still does.

One of the nice things about business protocol is that it's fairly straight forward. Efficiency is the operative idea, and mutual respect underscores everything. Equal status requires equal treatment — and pay. The rules of rank and age are virtually inviolate. Your sex has nothing to do with it.

Business etiquette is like a current that sweeps away any murky confusion. At the bottom it attempts to exclude the notion of gender. It isn't a perfect system, of course, but it's workable and getting better. The message for men is: *Forget sexual distinctions. Don't shy away from being critical with women if criticism is called for. Call it the way it is.*

There are practical and legal reasons to adopt such a policy. A failure (or lack of courage) to be even-handed wastes talent and, if the situation is volatile, may well wind up in court. Sex discrimination suits are as commonplace as fender-benders. This may be an unbalanced situation, fraught with all kinds of unfairness, but it's a real-world problem that men need to cope with. Surely there's no need to ask for big time trouble when a little attitude adjustment is all that's needed.

The social climate outside the office remains unsettled. Man/woman relations are still in flux; of course they always have been, and probably will remain touch-and-go for the foreseeable future. But legal precedents and social change have combined to "sanitize" the workplace. The corporate culture is the epitome of today's unisex lifestyles, or at least such is the intent. As far as we're concerned, it's a blessing for both sexes.

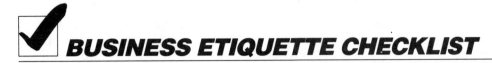

BUSINESS ETIQUETTE CHECKLIST

We've discussed briefly the general outlines of male/female on-the-job etiquette. This checklist gets to the specifics, the basics. With the concept of a non-genderized workplace as a starting point, the following tips of the trade are offered:

☐ **Helping with a coat or jacket:** Women help men and vice- versa. It's really a matter of who needs the assistance at any given moment.

☐ **Opening and closing doors:** If a man and woman arrive simultaneously at the door, the general rule is that the person with the least baggage gets the door. If you know the woman well enough to allow your traditional gentlemanly instincts to take over, it's okay to play doorman. She probably won't be offended. If you have doubts, play it safe. However, if you hold a door for a woman and she views it as an insult, don't worry about it; something's missing from her background, and that isn't your responsibility.

☐ **Business dining;** This one is simple. The one who does the inviting pays. There's no reason to deviate from the rule; after all, you've been invited for professional reasons or because you're a colleague, not just because you're a nice guy.

☐ **Introductions:** Higher positions are introduced to lower. However, there are cases where a customer would be more important than anyone in your organization at introduction time. Use your judgment to determine who is most important.

☐ **The old devil, touching:** Aside from a sincere, firm handshake, touching is definitely out. Eye contact is important, but men need to make that contact purely objective no matter how attractive your female colleague may be. In other words, keep a cool eye at all times. If you've known or worked closely with a woman there's always a possibility of an affectionate touch on the arm or hand. Yet this remains explosive territory. Think about it from the female point-of-view and ask yourself what you'd think if a woman workmate touched you. It's easy to see how someone might leap to the wrong conclusion.

☐ **Opening and closing car doors:** If the parties arrive together and it's convenient, men may get the door for a woman with little risk of offense. However, today's woman has no reason to expect a man to open and close car doors in a business setting. When exiting the car, most women will open her door and won't sit there waiting for assistance.

☐ **Smoking:** You should refrain in business situations, especially with cigarettes, which carry all sorts of unpleasant connotations. This rule is true for either sex. During a break or after hours the rules change and social protocol prevails. It's always important to ask companions if they mind your smoking.

☐ **Health talk:** In a business setting, both women and men will assume you're healthy and fit; otherwise, you wouldn't be there. If you feel out of sorts, do everything possible to cover up. If someone else is complaining, don't let it be an invitation to do the same. Anyone who insists on talking about his or her health at a business session is out of line. Listen politely, then move on.

☐ **Discussions of family or other loved ones:** What would you think if a female client suddenly made inquiries about your marriage or asked a lot of questions about your wife or fiance? You'd probably think it odd at best, nosey at worst, and you'd wonder about her sense of privacy. If a woman knows you're married or engaged it's okay to answer a few light questions. But only a few. Confine such conversation to social situations.

☐ **Criticizing:** Many men still feel shy about criticizing women. For some reason they tend to revert back to their traditional upbringing and think thoughts of the "weaker sex." Unfortunately this is a self-defeating attitude. If you see flaws in the reasoning or plans of a female colleague you owe it to her — and yourself! — to point them out. Ideas shouldn't be subject to sexual differences; ideas often equal profits, and profits don't take well to wimps. Call it as you see it.

☐ **Personal compliments:** Believe it or not, it's still in good taste to offer a deserved compliment on a woman's appearance or the way she handles a business matter. You need to be very judicious about the former (better know the woman you're complimenting) and open about the latter. Refrain from personal references toward a woman business associate you've just met. Your kindness is too easy to misconstrue, and it isn't worth the risk.

CHAPTER TEN

DINING FOR DOLLARS:

Breaking Bread Business Style

"**M**ost of the deals cut in this country are locked-up between 7 a.m. and noon," says New York-based management consultant Tom Pettibone. "The next most critical time is between 5 p.m. and about 9 p.m. That's when a lot of business people get together with possible clients, at dinner."

Pettibone suggests that breaking bread has become a standard ritual in doing business, so much so that the social aspects of breakfast, lunch, and dinner are merely a cover for the real purpose of these repasts — making money!

"I have to be as sharp in a restaurant as I would be facing a board of directors. Maybe even sharper," he says. "At least in a conference room I don't have to worry about spilling the soup."

Pettibone is part of the upswing in the importance of breaking bread business-style. Even with new tax laws in place that severely limit what the Internal Revenue Service calls "the three-martini business lunch," dining for dollars continues unabated. One reason may be that professionals want insight on the "whole person" they're doing business with, and the semi-social ambience of the business meal goes a long way in revealing one's ability to carry off a triple-A job of image maintenance.

It's not enough these days to look great and have professional credentials. You need social skills, too. The test often takes place over a white linen table cloth in an executive bistro.

Peggy Whedon, co-author (with John Kidner) of *Dining in the Great Embassies*, says the emphasis on executive social grace grew out of the standard practices of international trade and diplomacy.

"For generations, foreign policy has been made — or sounded out — at embassy dinners," says Whedon, who is a former producer of NBC's "This Week With David Brinkley." "People wonder why these are such elaborate affairs. The answer is that it's part of the cost of doing business on an international scale."

Whether it's foreign or domestic business you're doing, breaking bread for dollars is an art no executive can do without. It's an indispensible facet of your total image, which is why we're including it here.

Dualing Alarm Clocks: The Executive Breakfast

Few challenges are more awesome than a pre-dawn breakfast meeting called by the boss. It's designed to test your endurance, to catch a glimpse of you at a time when you might be most vulnerable to an inadvertent slip-up. Naturally, there's business at-hand; we're not implying that a pre-dawn curtain call is a sadistic game in the corporation's 24-hour-a-day life cycle. On the contrary, it's a way to add valuable hours to any project. And it works. Show us an executive who's up before dawn and, nine out of 10 times, we'll show you a success.

Training for Dualing Alarm Clocks

The boss has called a breakfast meeting for 6:30 a.m., a half-hour before you normally open your eyes. He or she wants a tactical plan for a meeting later that day with the owners of ABC Corporation, which your company is hoping to purchase. Obviously you'll need to be in high gear long before the V-8 is served. How do you prepare?

The first step begins the night before the meeting. Get all the necessary paperwork done; you don't want to be dotting "i's" and crossing "t's" by dawn's early light. Besides, you'll need those early pre-meeting hours to get your heart pumping.

It helps to place your papers and reports in well-marked folders. Go over each before turning in. If there are any last minute items that need attention, now's the time to handle them.

Don't worry about the sleep you're going to miss. Unless you're one of those people who needs a full eight hours, why try to force your natural cycle? Forcing it leads to high anxiety, a lot of tossing and turning, and a whipped countenance in the morning. Most men are fit enough to handle a night of minimal sleep (or none at all) and still be sufficiently alert in the morning to get through a day at the office.

Lay out your complete wardrobe the night before. Fumbling in a dark closet isn't a lot of fun, and there's always a risk of selecting the wrong items. If you're a veteran, remember your happy days in boot camp when you knew exactly what the uniform of the day would be. Take the same approach in dressing for the business breakfast.

Be out of bed with time to spare; you're going to need it. You'll be getting into high gear very quickly, and your motor may be a little balky when you wake up. You know in advance that the boss will be pumping adrenalin at a rate of 12 pints a second, and you'll want to keep the pace.

If you need a fresh cup of coffee to start the day, have it *before* you hit the road. You don't want to wait until the actual breakfast for that first slug of caffeine. For all you know, some health-conscious colleague — probably the boss — will have a pallid decaffeinated brew on hand. If you're really groggy, try a Coke or Pepsi instead of coffee. Soft drinks generally have more caffeine in them. A new favorite is Jolt Cola, which boasts "all the sugar and twice the caffeine" as ordinary soft drinks. "Jolt" is a favorite for early-rising construction workers, so you know it really works.

Turn on the TV or radio to catch the news. It's a good idea to check on what's been happening in that darkened world outside your window. If the morning paper has been delivered, read the front page and the business section. There may be an item of interest that will give you an extra edge at the meeting. If so, great. If not, at least you've got your mind working. It's a proven form of cerebral sit-ups.

Do a light physical workout before you hit the shower. No matter how fuzzy you may feel, a workout will push you through the fog. Don't overdo it. You'd be surprised how many fitness-oriented executives go too far and nod out during the meeting. No matter how fit you are, the combination of an early hour and physical exertion poses this threat.

Eat something light before you leave home or on the way to work. It isn't a great idea to show up with a ravenous appetite. Besides, the fare typically served at these bouts of dualing alarm clocks isn't what you'd want to order for yourself. So get the energy food before you arrive.

Once on the scene, be especially cautious of messy items like jelly donuts or sunny-side-up eggs. These seem to have a sneaky way of jumping right onto your tie. Play it safe, eat only those items that are easy to handle.

Dressing Tips for Early A.M.

Sunrise is a time for very conservative clothing. Your outfit should be easy and comfortable; it should speak softly and not butt in. A gray or navy suit is a pick. You may want to avoid a white shirt. White has a lot of dazzle at sunrise. A blue shirt is less formal.

Make sure that your tie is conservative, too. It isn't a good idea to jar your colleagues awake with fire engine red or "yum-yum" yellow.

When it's your turn to make a report or ask questions, try to frame your ideas simply; nothing argumentative unless absolutely necessary. Remember boot camp and your drill instructor, and do exactly the opposite.

No matter how challenging the hour, these basic tips will help you be a winner at dualing alarm clocks.

The Business Lunch

Despite the popularity of the lunchtime fitness workout, the ritual of "doing lunch" for dollars remains a standard practice.

Thankfully, the business lunch is less demanding than dualing alarm clocks. Most of the time it's an enjoyable event, though its context keeps it from being entirely relaxing. In some circles (publishing and advertising, for example) it's an absolute imperative for successful business relationships. Once the exclusive domain of upper management, lunching for dollars is now democratically realigned so that everyone from the mailroom to the boardroom is expected to participate at one time or another. The following tips will help you make the most of it while projecting a smooth, efficient image:

● **Invitations:** If you're the one doing the inviting, give your guests 48 hours notice. Call the restaurant well ahead of time and make the reservation in your name and the name of your company. Let them know how many will be in your party. If you expect to do some serious talking, ask for a table that's out of the way; roomy enough to accommodate paperwork, if any. If you intend to pay with a credit card make sure the restaurant honors your particular form of plastic. Keep cash on hand, too, just in case there's a slip-up.

● **Arrive early:** Give yourself a 15 minute cushion. Check in with the *maitre d'*. Recheck your reservations: "Yes, it's the Smith party of four, and we need a table out of traffic. Business, you know . . . " While you're waiting, check over the menu and the wine list, and let the *maitre d'* take an impression of your credit card, since you're paying. Make sure the check is handed directly to you. Wait in the lobby to greet your guests. If there is no lobby, proceed to the table. Seat yourself facing the entrance so you can see guests arrive. If documents are to be passed around, seat your guests so that the senior person is on your right.

This insures that the most important person sees the papers first. Place the documents neatly beside you, with your briefcase stowed beneath the table.

- **"Twelve o' clocktails":** To drink or not to drink? This, indeed, is the question. Ask your guests if they'd like a pre- lunch drink. If no one wants alcohol, you should abstain, too. If only one guest wants a drink it's okay to join in as long as you stick to wine or beer. No hard stuff. Suggesting a pony glass of champagne is usually a winner. Those who accept won't be viewed as heavy mid-day drinkers by those who decline. It's amazing how that little pony of champagne cuts across all barriers to nullify objections. Whatever happens, *don't be the only drinker at the table,* and under no circumstances should you push alcohol: "It's okay, a little won't hurt . . . " You may be talking to a recovering problem drinker.

- **Proper form:** Place the napkin in your lap as soon as you're seated. If you need to leave the table for any reason, place the napkin to the left of your plate and replace it on your lap as soon as you return. Exact etiquette forbids tucking the napkin under your belt, but practical concerns dictate otherwise. Elbows are off the table while eating, but it's okay to rest your forearms there between courses. When eating, bring the food to your mouth — not mouth to food. No smoking during meals (unless you're in Russia, where this is common practice). After a meal, smoke only if you gracefully gain permission from others at the table. If possible, abstain.

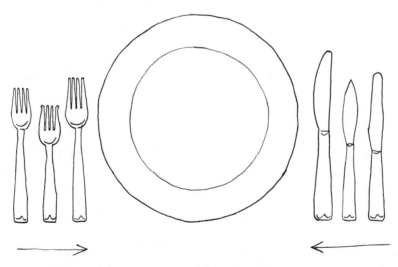

Use utensils from the outside and work your way inward.

Extra Tips for the Business Lunch Host

- Wait for your guests to order before making your selections.
- Allow guests to read the menu in silence. If you know the restaurant,

you may make suggestions. *Do not suggest anything unless you've tried it personally.*

● Before getting down to business, relax your guests with small talk. No jokes, please! Especially no ethnic humor!

● Don't allow your important business conversation to be interrupted by the menu coming or the dishes being cleared away. You can arrange a series of signals through the *maitre d'* ahead of time.

● If you need to excuse yourself, simply say, "excuse me, please." No need to mention why.

● No matter how bad the food or service, never make a scene. You can vocalize your gripes with the restaurant later, out of earshot.

● Watch time and keep the meeting on schedule. It's up to you to make first sign of ending lunch meeting to return to office.

The Business Dinner

Except that the late hour gives it a slightly more formal ambience, the rules of the business dinner are similar to those generally practiced at lunch. Dress, however, should be a cut or two above what you'd wear earlier in the day.

To get into the swing of the evening, you may wish to add a solid silk necktie and a white shirt with French cuffs. The idea is to avoid looking as if you've just switched off the lights at the office and hurried over to make your dinner appointment, even if this is precisely what you've done. This is especially important for small functions after work. Social evenings demand a more dressed up look. Appropriate dress for the occasion continues to be an important part of your presentation. Bring the extras to the office and make the switch before leaving. You might also take a reading on your "five o'clock shadow." If late in the day you bear an uncanny resemblance to Richard Nixon, use the razor you've stowed in your desk to freshen up. Give your shoes a quick buffing, and you're off!

Even if, as the TV ads proclaim, "the night belongs to Michelob" (and other wet delights), your professional image requires that you be extra conservative in the drinking department. One drink before dinner is acceptable; the outside limit is two. Under no circumstances should you cajole others into drinking. If everyone is the group is on the wagon for the evening, common sense and propriety demands that you join them.

If you're the host, wait until the others have ordered their meals before you do. Take a cue from your guests. If they're eating lightly, so should you. Keeping everyone waiting while you consume a multi-course meal is no way to ingratiate yourself. Grab a snack at home if you're still hungry later on.

Condiments and butter that are shared require certain considerations by the host. Always pass them to your guests first. When they come your way, place a small amount on your plate. Break your bread or dinner roll in small pieces and butter it one bite at a time. This advice may sound a bit finicky, but it's correct form.

Perhaps you want to toast one or all of your guests. Fine — but keep it under three minutes. Most psychologists will tell you that the average attention span is slightly less than 20 seconds. Toasts need to be framed with a merciful understanding of human limits.

In greeting people it's pretty much a matter of form over substance, so there's no need to be anything but cheerful and polite. When greeting someone in your home, office, or at restaurant, correct form is to rise, smile, shake hands, mention your name (if it's someone new), and make a point of mentioning the guest's name. Make your introductions to the other guests. It helps to tell a tiny bit about the person you're introducing. "Jim, meet Bill. He's the guy who makes up those terrific brochures for us..." A small touch will personalize and lighten what otherwise may be a too-formal scene. If you wish to keep an air of formality to the proceedings, use official titles instead of an off-the-cuff description of what a person does professionally.

Strange Sounding Names: Wine Lists

Wine has become very popular in the U.S. It's light, it's bright. Fitness folks think it's less caloric than most other alcohol (that's a myth, but so what!), and it fits in nicely with the image professionals hope to maintain.

However, this brings us to a challenge that almost every mobile male must face — *knowing and understanding wines!* Specifically, it means deciphering extensive wine lists. Even before they're old enough to drink, young men understand the chore they face. They know that becoming familiar with wine lists is tougher than learning Greek!

Not so when it comes to wine. Wine, it seems, is infinite. How can any one human being ever get to know — let alone love — even a tiny fraction of what's available?

Homework is the key, which isn't so bad, really. There are worse things than tasting wines and deciding which are best for your style. Of course a real scholar goes a step beyond and figures out which wines go best with different personalities. This, indeed, is considered a true mark of achievement.

Some restaurants use hard sell when they hand you a wine list. They're not terribly subtle about it, either. No one in his right mind is going to select the cheapest item on the list, particularly if there are guests. Nor can you expect to get by with a mid-priced dark horse. Unless you know your wines first-hand, you have no choice but to be on the pricey side. Price, restaurant owners know, is the best bluff. It goes with the axiom that says he (or she) who doesn't know wines will pay dearly to learn.

If you don't already have a working knowledge of wines, it makes sense to do something about it. In the meantime, these simple guidelines may help:

● **Red wines:** Complement red meat, game, and pasta. Some people say red wines go to the head faster than white varieties. With spicy seafood or pasta, red wine is often a good choice.

● **White wines:** Dry whites are typically ordered with fish or poultry. Sweet whites are best with desserts. Whites are generally less caloric than reds.

● **Champagne:** A no-miss selection. It goes with everything. Everyone knows what it tastes like and how it feels.

● **Breaking rules:** Today people mix and match wines with all sorts of foods. Nowhere it is absolutely decreed that red goes with red meat, white with fish. If someone is nervey enough to be critical of you for breaking the "rules" (such as they are) that person probably knows less about wine than you do!

It isn't gauche to ask your guests which wines they prefer. The gesture is sensible, polite, and it circumvents having to put on a show. Some people can't drink reds because they're allergic to them, so asking will avoid a "dining-out malpractice suit" and leave you looking like the man for whom the word "culture" was named.

The 'Power Tea'

What on earth is a "Power Tea?"

It's one of the trendiest new trends, modeled approximately after the traditional British event, with the special American corporate touch — "power" added.

The Power Tea satisfies many needs. It provides a mid-afternoon break for those who work out instead of lunching (the teas are typically held between 4 p.m. and 6 p.m.). While some provide light wine, most are non-alcoholic. The food is generally on the light side: scones, finger snacks, watercress, paper-thin wafers — the expected low-calorie spread served by health-conscious men and women on the way up.

The power part goes directly to the corporate identity of the teas. You can expect to meet your professional peers at these affairs, which may be held at someone's office, home, or in the "fern bars" of major metropolitan cities.

If you haven't yet been invited to a "Power Tea," be patient; sooner or later, you'll be on someone's list. It's a new and refreshing way to do business.

BEING CONFIDENT
OF WHAT TO REACH FOR AND WHEN

Rest position

Finished position

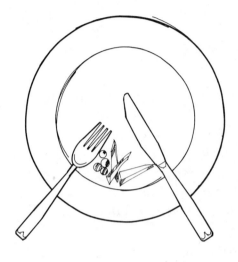
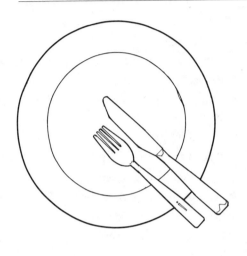

There is a wide array of silverware to encounter

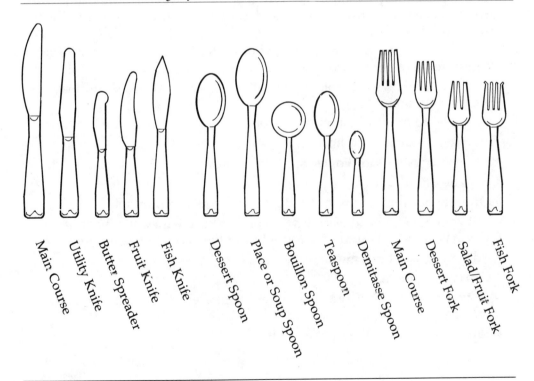

Main Course

Utility Knife

Butter Spreader

Fruit Knife

Fish Knife

Dessert Spoon

Place or Soup Spoon

Bouillon Spoon

Teaspoon

Demitasse Spoon

Main Course

Dessert Fork

Salad/Fruit Fork

Fish Fork

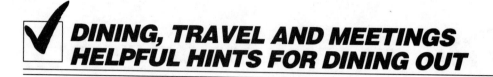

DINING, TRAVEL AND MEETINGS
HELPFUL HINTS FOR DINING OUT

☐ Send or answer invitations within 48 hours.

☐ Book reservations in advance.

☐ Arrive early.

- Give names of expected guests to *maitre d'*.
- Pre-select or look over wine list.
- Wait in lobby and greet guests; if lobby is not large enough, proceed to table.
- Stand as guests arrive and for introduction.
- Arrange seating, keeping in mind personalities and business.

☐ **If you are the guest:**

- Arrive no later than 10 to 15 minutes after planned time.
- No need to bring gift, send gift home or thank you next day.

☐ Leave coats, briefcase, etc., in checkroom.

☐ Do not have more than one drink before dinner.

☐ Seating: Sit so host can see door.

☐ Place napkin on lap as soon as seated. If you must leave before end for any reason, place napkin to left of plate and replace as soon as you return. Do not tuck napkin into belt.

☐ Do not put any briefcase, package, etc. on table. If work must be done during dinner, remove papers from briefcase.

☐ Do not put elbows on table while eating. Between courses you may rest forearms on table.

☐ Bring food to mouth, not mouth to food.

☐ **Ordering if you are the host:**

- Make suggestions and/or recommendations.
- Let guests order first.
- Order appetizer if anyone else does so they feel comfortable.
- Tell your guests ahead of time if you plan to have wine and what selections you have made. You can wait to select until everyone has ordered.

☐ **Ordering if you are a guest:**

- Order from menu.
- If you are the only one having an appetizer or hors d'oeuvres, you may cancel.
- Use flatware according to placemat.

- Bread and butter - put on bread and butter plate, break roll into small pieces as needed.
- If no bread and butter plate, put on table next to forks, this is correct continental style.
- Use correct resting position and finished position for cutlery.
- Do not smoke during dinner, always ask after dinner.
- Place napkin on left side when finished. Do not fold, place neatly.
- Guest of honor should be first to leave.
- Must send thank you or call next day.
- Tipping - 15-20% for dinner
  Wine steward (10% of wine bill)
  Maitre d' (optional, flat fee)

☐ Helpful Hints for Difficult Food

- Soup: scoop away from you.
- Pasta: cut flat pasta, swirl string pasta.
- Shrimp Cocktail: do not try to cut shrimp, use cocktail fork and take bites.
- Fruit: use knife and fork.
- Clams, oysters: hold shell with hand and eat with cocktail fork, do not stack shells.
- Chicken or fowl: do not use fingers, cut or pull segment off and then cut in bite-sized pieces.
- Fish with bones: cut off tail and head, cut along backbone, fold back meat, remove whole skeleton and set aside before starting to eat.

✔ DINING FOR DOLLARS CHECKLIST

Professional know-how and social graces are intermingled to a degree unheard of in the 1950's and early 1960's, when the "man in the gray flannel suit" was a hard-driving, ambitious "corporation man" who could down every martini in Bombay. Today men still wear gray flannel, but they're more likely to work for a dozen outfits before settling into blissful entrepreneurship. They drink and eat less; they socialize more. The women in their lives work, too — outside the kitchen. They're making peace with a unisex culture and sharpening their *savoir-faire*. One of the great tests for the new male involves breaking bread — and at the same time making big bucks. This checklist will help you do it in style.

☐ **Train for "dualing alarm clocks" — the executive breakfast:** Prepare all papers the night before. Give yourself plenty of time to wake up, catch the news on T.V. or on the front page, do a light workout and have your first cup of coffee. Have some light energy food before you arrive. The typical executive breakfast goes mostly uneaten.

☐ **Beware of messy foods:** Jelly doughnuts were made to squirt on your early morning necktie. Sunny-side-up eggs are equally pernicious. The safest thing at the executive breakfast is the toast — but without those squishy plastic jelly prewraps.

☐ **Dress down:** The uniform for "dualing alarm clocks" is conservative. A gray or navy suit and a very hushed tie with a blue or pastel shirt works well in this setting. This time of the morning is definitely quiet; help keep it that way.

☐ **Learn to live with (and love!) the executive lunch:** It's going to be a way of life for you. Remember, it's business. Also remember that good table manners help the bottom line. No hard charging and no hard sells. You'll accomplish more with your excellent social skills.

☐ **Plan ahead:** If you're the host, give guests 48 hours notice. Book reservations in advance and make sure you get the bill. If there are documents, put the senior person on your right so that he or she can read them first. Book a table out of the flow of traffic, and tell the maitre d' to watch your signals. You don't want waiters breaking in during a business discussion.

☐ **Arrive early:** Check the scene, the menu, the wine list. Wait in the lobby for your guests. If there's no lobby proceed to the table. Stand and greet each guest, with all the appropriate introductions.

☐ **Allow guests to give you clues:** If they're eating light, follow suit. If they don't want alcohol, order coffee or a soft drink for yourself. Never insist on alcohol for anyone; you may be cajoling a recovering problem drinker. You might order a light wine or a pony glass of champagne if the guests say they'd enjoy it. Stay away from the hard stuff.

☐ **Proper form is everything:** If you don't already know how to use the utensils, or if you're vague on etiquette generally, do a little research at the public library or take an etiquette course. You'll be surprised how simple and convenient good table manners can be.

☐ **Make only judicious suggestions from the menu:** If you haven't tried it, don't knock it and don't plug it!

☐ **Think placid:** No matter what happens — even if soup is spilled in your lap by your server — stay cool. If you have complaints (or cleaning bills) take them up after your guests have departed.

☐ **Executive dinners call for a dash of elegance:** Wear a solid silk tie and a clean shirt. If you don't have time to run home and freshen up, do it before you leave the office. You may be in a terrible rush, but you won't look it. As the TV ad suggests, "Never let 'em see you sweat!"

☐ **Make up your mind to learn something about wines:** It's a male prerequisite, and one of the easiest ways to impress others. If you're unsure about the selection, ask your guests what they'd enjoy. You'll never go wrong ordering wine by special request. If you and your guests draw a blank, go for champagne. It goes with anything.

☐ **Remember the "Power Tea":** If you haven't been invited yet, you surely will be. It's a light, typically non-alcoholic occasion, and the business side of things will certainly be there with the watercress and Perrier.

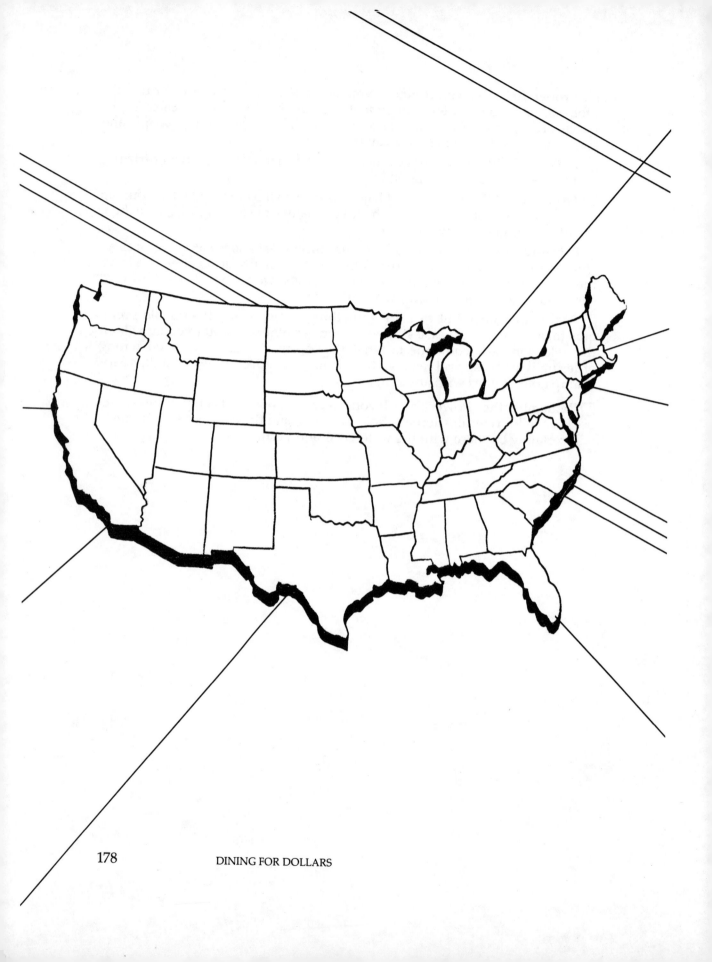

178   DINING FOR DOLLARS

CHAPTER ELEVEN
•••

UP, UP
AND AWAY

Traveling in Style and Comfort

Pooser's Law of Success and Motion: The degree of one's success and upward mobility is directly proportional to the amount of time spent dashing through airports, hopping on and off jet planes, and checking into hotels at distant ports of call!

Let's face it. The most successful executives are constantly on the go. As a matter of fact, there are "head- hunters" out there who will tell you that if you're not soaring about the clouds 50% of the time on route to do business, you're probably overdue for a job switch.

I can't vouch for the precise amount of travel time it takes to equal success nor can I make sweeping generalizations about sky-bound executives. But I can tell you about my own experiences.

Between 1986 and 1987, I logged more than 200,000 air miles while my business doubled in volume. Looking ahead, I see even more blue sky, which happens to coincide with a projected growth in Accolade's bottom line.

It would be okay if all I — or you — had to do was fly. Flying, after all, is a magical, often exciting experience, which borders on adventure while introducing us to new faces and places. But flying isn't enough in today's business world. It's coming back down to earth that presents us with a thousand-and-one unspeakable fortunes. There's luggage, lost and found; desk clerks who seem to have lost your hotel reservations; taxi drivers who, when you tell them where you want to go, reply in any language but English that no such address exists in that town.

There are obligatory breakfasts across time zones when your body is crying out for dinner, and cities, such as Moscow, where there isn't a drop of coffee or a snack to be had after 10 o'clock. There are cities where at 3:00 in the morning your hosts insist on sushi and the spiciest ginger on earth. Within 24 hours, you can be stuffed, starved, sleepy, hyperactive, and wondering if privacy has been outlawed!

Oh, yes, the spoils of success. You either accept them or drop out, or fly away to a commune in Oregon where business travel is strictly for squares. Indeed, this seems to be the choice these days with precious little compromise in between. It appears that the more valuable you are to your family, company, country, the more you'll need to love and live with the trying side of success — travel.

Traveling Women And Men

Of course, it's slightly different for women. At the risk of sounding sexist, I believe men have a slightly easier go of it. Men are typically bigger, stronger, more assertive and better equipped to handle the rigors of the road. This isn't to say that men don't face challenges and inconveniences; they do, in large, quelling doses. At airports all over the world I have seen men fit enough to handle a lineman's spot in the National Football League reduced to pleading for relief after a week on the road. I have watched porters happily assist women while men, weary and disheveled, are neglected. Chivalry may not be dead, but these poor men seem to be closer by the minute.

Such situations play havoc with the real business at hand. Travel, after all, is a means, not an end, and showing up road-weary and exhausted at a client's office is bad news no matter what the reason.

There isn't any way I know of to make travel seem like a magic carpet ride. But I do know from hard experience the ways and means to ease the most wearisome aspects of travel in our go-go, international, and domestic business community.

Enduring the Unbelievable

Here are some experiences I was forced to endure. As is often the case, in retrospect, they are funny — they were not at the time. Hopefully they will not be experienced again.

● I arrived in my hotel after 20 hours of continuous travel. None of my flights served a meal and I was subsequently forced to endure a steady diet of flat cokes and peanuts softened with the delectable taste of chemical preservatives.

After learning that the hotel restaurant was closed and that room service was no longer available, I retired to my room and enjoyed the culinary delights purchased from the hotel's vending machines. *Moral of the story:* Only select hotels providing twenty-four hour room service. Bring snacks of fruit or healthfood bars along for emergencies.

● I arrived in Sydney, Australia after 30 hours of travel at 6:00 A.M. local time. In this case, both room service and the hotel's restaurant were open — however — my room would not be ready until 1:00 P.M. In this case I was not hungry, for the succulent boiled meat and microwaved succotash served on the flight more than satisfied my quivering tastebuds. All I wanted was a hot shower and a place to get horizontal. Nodding off in the hotel lobby in fermenting clothes does not an executive image make. *Moral of the story:* It is worth the money to book an extra day to avoid this type of complication.

● On a relatively short trip within the United States, I arrived at my hotel with what I thought was plenty of time to ready myself for a meeting. All that I needed was the hotel laundry service to get the wrinkles out of the clothes I had laid out. I am sure that they would have done this with the utmost courtesy and efficiency except for the fact that this hotel had no laundry service. In my room, I found myself in my weakness in the middle of what seemed to be an experiment to determine how badly I could scald myself with my travel iron. Fortunately, although my clothes still looked wrinkled, I was sweating profusely from the iron's steam. This did allow my facial mask to work quite well. *Moral of the story:* check ahead on laundry service as well as other necessities.

● The time: twenty minutes before my scheduled morning meeting. The place: New York City. The situation: a torrential downpour and no taxi stand in front of my hotel. My choices: walk ten blocks to the meeting and hope to get a cab on the way or skip the meeting and go back to bed. The last choice, although feasible, was not to my long-term benefit. *Moral of the story:* The "wet" look is not in. Book a hired car or taxi the night before.

Helpful Hints for a Pleasant Journey

Below are some tips that have worked for me. With a little ingenuity and discipline you can apply them to make life on the wing a bit more civilized no matter where you have to go in this frantic world.

● Have secretary book airline reservations in advance — use corporate discounts — including your seat selection. Ask if meals will be served. Order any special meals ahead. Vegetarian meals are light and a nice change for long flights.

● Bring health food bar, fruit, or crackers for emergency delays.

● Allow more than one hour between flights if stopping at busy airport (Atlanta, Chicago, Washington, D.C., etc.)

● Arrive the night before for important early morning meetings.

- If possible, do not check bags (see packing tips below). Use garment bag and briefcase.
- Limit alcohol on long flights, suggestion - mix fruit juice and wine. Drink extra water, juice, etc. Alcohol adds to dehydration.
- Book hotel near meetings and not at airport regardless of late arrival. It is easier and safer to be on time in the morning.
- Take taxi from airport. If weather is bad, arrange for hired car at airport. This is often only $10-15 more but can save hours.
- Check hotel facilities and services ahead:
  - 24-hour room service (some hotels stop room service at 11:00 p.m. This is not helpful if you arrive after 11:00 and hungry)
  - dry cleaning
  - restaurant services - if reservations are necessary
  - taxi availability for early morning
  - secretarial services
  - concierge
  - ask about room location - to assure quiet
    - near elevator?
    - street side?
    - construction?

✓ TRAVEL PLANNER

☐ **To plan your clothing needs, determine:**
- *Climate:* • Chicago in January? • Tropics.
- *Nature of trip:* • Business, • Pleasure, • Combination.
- *Length of trip and activities?* • How many days? • Meetings? • Sightseeing? • Elegant evenings, etc.?
- *Itinerary?* • Overnight only? • Complicated transfers?
- *Who will you be with?* • Will you be in the same place with the same people? If you will be in different places or with different people, you will need fewer clothing items.

☐ **Selecting Clothing for a Trip**

This is a sample wardrobe for one-week business trip.
- 2 suits: navy and gray
- Sports coat and slacks (you may want to travel in them)
- 5 shirts: white and blue
- 5 ties
- Pair black lace up shoes
- Extra pair of sport shoes: loafers
- Dark leather belt
- 5 pair of socks
- Raincoat/trench coat
- Sweater, cap and gloves for cold weather
- Exercise, swim, or jogging wear

☐ **Men Travel kit**
- Shaving kit, hair brush, hair dryer, shampoo/spray
- Toothbrush, toothpaste
- Deodorant, miscellaneous medicine
- Lint brush, stick spot remover, travel sewing kit
- Travel alarm clock
- Umbrella
- Name and address book
- Steamer/iron
- AC/DC adapter

✔ TRAVELING IN STYLE AND COMFORT CHECKLIST

Executives today are constantly on the go. In spite of the aura of excitement when traveling to new and different places, inevitable inconveniences are thrown out in paths.

Both men and women are subject to the challenges when traveling. In some ways men have it worse — the "fair damsel" message works to get help and assistance when none is available to the disheveled gentleman. This adds to the importance of "planning ahead."

☐ **Book airline reservations including seat selection and special meals ahead —** bring snacks along for emergencies.

☐ Allow sufficient time for flight connections and transportation from airport to hotel to meeting.

☐ Check hotel facilities ahead including restaurant and room service hours, laundry, secretarial services, renovation and construction on premises.

☐ Consider climate, length of trip, and itinerary and pack accordingly. Bring **appropriate** clothes for different functions.

☐

WHERE YOU'RE HEADED

In Tomorrow's New Age

Gaze into your crystal ball and project your image into the Shining New Age of the Year 2000. What do you see there? What will the world be like and how will you fit in?

If the pundits are correct, you may be adjusting to a whole new profession in the so-called "Information Age." It may even be your second or third career adjustment, with more to come. Not a terribly settling prospect, I admit, but perhaps unavoidable as time and distance shrink, populations shift, new socio-economic demands tug at our wallets, and the relatively cozy world we took to bed last night comes up with a surprising (though not necessarily pleasing) new look at dawn's early light.

I'm not suggesting that all change is disorienting or threatening. It depends on whose up and whose not, whose in or out, and how well you're able to shift gears at the right time. Chances are better than ever that in a few years you'll be tougher, wiser, more sophisticated, better prepared to shape your destiny.

If the information age brings career adjustments, it also promises more travel, new ways of relating to men and women in the geo-political sphere. In the years ahead we'll be more international, probably ordering Japanese and Chinese cuisine in the native languages. And when it comes to women, be assured that today's social "revolution" won't end.

It probably never will, despite new laws and moves that redefine sexual equality. For example, more than a half century ago, the late H.L. Mencken, with typically caustic sarcasm, declared that a gentlemen "is one who never strikes a woman without provocation." Today, *Cosmopolitan* magazine's editor-

-in-chief, Helen Gurley Brown, responded with equal absurdity that a lady "no doubt is one who never supplies the provocation!" So much for progress!

But fashion — that is bound to change. Our whole system of free enterprise is based on it. Would this be America if we weren't induced to buy a new car every year, or move into a bigger home, or transform our sexual habits, or find new foods to microwave? Why should fashion be any different? If anything, those who dress us up or down will continue to put us through endless variations of what's in and/or out. Hemlines will be kicked up and down relative to the width of your neckties. Chic today will be klutsy tomorrow. "Moon threads" — fabrics spun in space stations — will replace wool and cotton only to be discarded next year for good old "earthwear."

What does all this mean in a world in which change is the only constant?

Perhaps the answer is in your mirror, in your reflection. You need to keep pace, of course, but who and what you are is the key to the future. Individual style doesn't fly away with frivolous fashion. It's the one constant, intangible as it may be. No matter what styles and fashions prevail at a given moment in history, the inner you makes decisions, holds to certain elements of good taste and personal presentation.

No Paris designer or Second Avenue cloth cutter is going to remake the essential you. No outrage of social maladjustment will transform your sense of fairness and balance. The ladies in your life will continue to challenge every move you make but chances are you won't go the Menckenesque route of wounded vanity covered by a cloth of "superman" insults. To summarize, you'll need flexibility. You'll hold fast to good taste, good manners, tolerance, understanding, a world view wide enough to accept diversity and change. You're going to be faithful to that mirror image because you know it's more than just you. It's a reflection of the future.

That is what a truly successful image is all about. It reflects today and hints at tomorrow. Like good taste in all ages, it's based on solid ground, uncompromised excellence, and perhaps the richest of all qualities: timelessness.

EPILOGUE

INDEX

●●

Celebrities

RESOURCES
●●

Always In Style Consultants Authorized to Conduct "Successful Image" Seminar

Mary Jane Barnes
953 "B" Street, **Virginia Beach, VA** 23451, (804) 428-4643

Bonny Barshay
499 E. Palmetto Park Road, #227, **Boca Raton, FL** 33432, (305) 392-8973

Kathryn Bryan
3800 Black Canyon Road, **Ft. Worth, TX** 76109, (817) 732-2170

Peg Carbone
11 Glen Arden Drive, **Fairfield, CT** 06430, (203) 255-7993

Keiko Couch
1928 Dartmoor Court, **Ft. Worth, TX** 76110, (817) 926-7675

Linda Denney
2305 26th Avenue, **Meridian, MS** 39305, (601) 693-6611

Jean Gaffney
12 Moore Lane, **Littleton, MA** 01460, (617) 486-8156

Liz Hale
1081 SE 172nd Street, #C, **Renton, WA** 98055, (206) 226-7412

Kathryn Kienke
888 8th Avenue, #5C, **New York, NY** 10019, (212) 974-0116

Maria Elena Leignadier
P.O. Box 5356, **Panama 5, Panama,** 64-3685

Barbara Lorenz
138 Christol Street, **Metuchen, NJ** 08840, (201) 548-0496

Saundra McCormick
714 Magnolia, **Modesto, CA** 95354, (209) 527-7480

Barbara McMeekin
2710 Broadway, **San Francisco, CA** 94115, (415) 567-9063

Joy Mahovich
4160 NW 99th Avenue, **Coral Springs, FL** 33065, (305) 752-5455

Nancy Matlin
514 Main Street, **Skokie, IL** 60077, (312) 677-6310

Angie Michael
2849 Lawrence Drive, **Falls Church, VA** 22042, (703) 560-3950

Bonnie Miller
Keeneland, Route 1, Box 10K, **Berryville, VA** 22611, (703) 955-4522

Helene Mills
930 California Avenue, Condo 301, **Santa Monica, CA** 90403, (213) 394-2282

Jane A. Murdoch
13806 Braddock Springs Rd. #A, **Centerville, VA** 22020, (703) 266-3073

Virginia Oakland
524 West Port Plaza, **St. Louis, MO** 63146, (314) 878-3494

Jackie Schluter
8 Belknap Lane, **Rumson, NJ** 07760, (201) 842-4120

Bettie Simpkins
134 Mine Lake Court, #100, **Raleigh, NC** 27615, (919) 847-5885

Kathy Skredvedt
3807 Timber Ridge Road, **Midlothian, VA** 23112, (804) 744-4460

Susan Straight
450 Maple Avenue, E., Suite 207, **Vienna, VA** 22108, (703) 938-4445

Elena De Virzi
6-14-95, **El Dorado, Panama** Rep de Pma, 61-5412

Barbara Warner
497 Clinton Avenue, **Toms River, NJ** 08753, (201) 240-6650

Mary Zimmerman
4539 Corrientes Circle, S., **Jacksonville, FL** 32217, (904) 739-3332

This listing is complete through September 1989. For the name of a consultant near you or our international consultant list call 1-800-EN-STYLE.

If you would like the name of the Always In Style consultant nearest you or information on how to become an Always In Style consultant please call 1-800-EN-STYLE.

ORDER FORM

Successful Style: A Man's Complete Guide To A Professional Image

☐ **Always In Style** Abridged swatches ($15.00)
Contains 18 fabric swatches, clear vinyl holder and wallet.

    ☐ Warm   ☐ Deep   ☐ Bright
    ☐ Cool   ☐ Light   ☐ Muted

☐ **Always In Style** Expanded swatches ($25.00)
Contains 48 fabric swatches, clear vinyl holder and wallet.

    ☐ Warm   ☐ Deep   ☐ Bright
    ☐ Cool   ☐ Light   ☐ Muted

☐ Please send me more information on your products.

☐ Please send me more information on your correspondence seminar programs:

    ☐ **SUCCESSFUL IMAGE SEMINAR** - This program includes: wardrobe planning based on individual body line and color analysis, body language and corporate etiquette for *men and women.*

    ☐ **WINNING IMAGE SEMINAR** - This program was developed especially for the hospitality industry. Customer service, grooming and body language are analyzed. Guidelines are provided to improve image, promote job pride and reduce turnover rates.

    ☐ **RETAIL CONNECTION SEMINAR** - A sales training seminar using **Always In Style** concepts to increase sales, repeat business and the professionalism and confidence of the sales staff.

Please fill out this coupon and mail with your check or money order payable to Accolade, Inc. to the following address: (Virginia residents add 4 1/2% sales tax)

      Always In Style
      c/o Accolade, Inc.
      311 Rivermont Avenue
      Suite B
      Lynchburg, Virginia 24504

Please send my order to:

Name _____

Address _____

_____

_____ Zip _____

N

RESOURCES